DANGEROUS SEA LIFE

OF THE WEST ATLANTIC, CARIBBEAN, AND GULF OF MEXICO

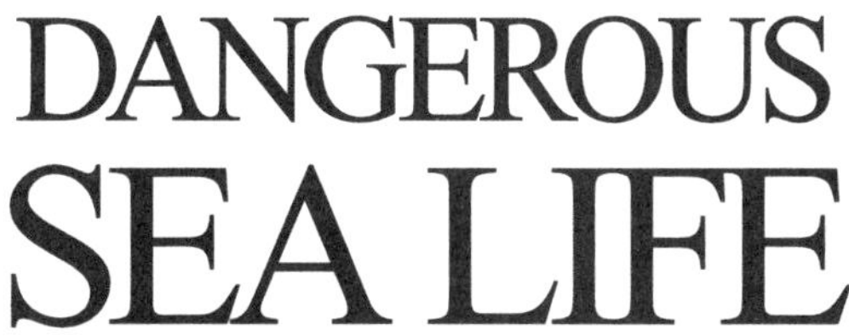

OF THE WEST ATLANTIC, CARIBBEAN,
AND GULF OF MEXICO

A Guide for Accident Prevention and First Aid

Edwin S. Iversen and Renate H. Skinner

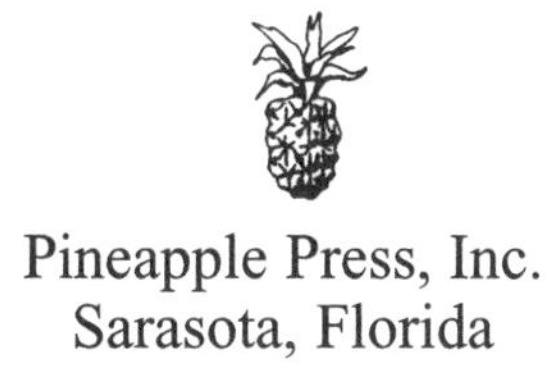

Pineapple Press, Inc.
Sarasota, Florida

Inquiries should be addressed to:

Pineapple Press, Inc.
P.O. Box 3889
Sarasota, Florida 34230

www.pineapplepress.com

Library of Congress Cataloging-in-Publication Data

Iversen, Edwin S.
Dangerous sea life of the west Atlantic, Caribbean, and Gulf of Mexico : a guide for accident prevention and first aid / Edwin S. Iversen and Renate H. Skinner.— 1st ed.
p. cm.
Includes bibliographical references and index.
ISBN-13: 978-1-56164-370-7 (pbk. : alk. paper)
ISBN-10: 1-56164-370-X (pbk. : alk. paper)
1. Dangerous marine animals. 2. First aid in illness and injury. I. Skinner, Renate H. II. Iversen, Edwin S. How to cope with dangerous sea life. III. Title.
QL100.I93 2006
616.9'8024—dc22

2006006650

First Edition
10 9 8 7 6 5 4 3 2 1

Design by Lisa McQuaid
Printed in the United States of America

Disclaimer
This publication is intended to acquaint the reader with the appearance and characteristics of dangerous sea life that can be encountered in the west Atlantic, the Caribbean, and the Gulf of Mexico. Neither publisher nor author claim that the list of organisms described herein is exhaustive of harmful organisms that may be encountered in the geographic region covered. This book should not be relied upon as a source of medical advice. The reader should seek immediate medical attention if an injury occurs.

For all marine enthusiasts: divers, fishermen, boaters, swimmers, and beachcombers

In Memoriam
Edwin Severin Iversen 1922–1999

Contents

Preface and Acknowledgments

The first version of our book was originally published in 1977 under the title *How to Cope with Dangerous Sea Life.* The present book is more comprehensive and helpful. Besides the latest practical knowledge on parasites, stings, and bites, it includes new sections and up-to-date information. We added several species, as well as a chapter on species that secrete toxic mucus, which is irritating to sensitive-skinned people. A new chapter addresses human interactions with large, potentially dangerous marine animals, and the caution swimmers should use when feeding, handling, or swimming with them.

The Atlantic coastal marine waters of the United States support extensive commercial and recreational fisheries. As the human population continues to grow, fishing is rapidly increasing, along with diving, boating, swimming, and other water-related activities. The substantial expenditures associated with sport fishing, boating, and SCUBA diving are valuable assets to the economy of coastal communities.

Our overall objective is to impart knowledge about potential harm from stinging, biting, or poisonous marine organisms, along with information on their parasites. We suggest ways to deal with problems which might develop, so that swimmers, boaters, divers, fishermen, and seafood lovers may find greater enjoyment of the sea along the western Atlantic coast, the Caribbean, and the Gulf of Mexico.

At the beginning of each chapter we provide a list of topics. We also advise on how to avoid harm from each dangerous group of species and offer information about prevention of possible problems before people are exposed to danger, or before consumers eat seafood which may be toxic to them. Readers who want more specific information will find publications listed for further reading at the end of each chapter. In Chapter 2 we include basic first aid summaries for victims of bites, stings, and other injuries. However, the main source concerning first aid should be a health professional.

The illustrations depict many well-known species along with some of the less common described in the text. Some are mentioned in more than one place in the book, since certain species may be aggressive and bite, as well as being toxic.

In the original 1977 manuscript we thanked Dr. Donald P. de Sylva and Robert C. Work, University of Miami, Rosenstiel School of Marine and Atmospheric Science, for their useful critique of the manuscript; Warren Zeiller and Jim La Tourrette, Miami Seaquarium, Dr. John Randall, Bernice Bishop Museum, Hawaii, and Frederick H. Berry, NMFS, Southeast Fisheries Center, for kindly providing photographs; and Jane Z. Iversen for editing.

In this updated book with new illustrations, we add our special thanks to Dr. Michael C. Schmale, Professor, University of Miami, Rosenstiel School of Marine and Atmospheric Science, for donating two of his personal underwater photographs, the octopus and stoplight parrotfish.

We especially thank Cecelia McCafferty for her diligent work on processing the manuscript and providing helpful suggestions toward making this a user-friendly book. We also owe many thanks to Adrienne Skinner for generously supplying office space and equipment.

INTRODUCTION

This guide describes potential dangers from certain marine life found in coastal areas of the western Atlantic of the United States from Maine to the Gulf of Mexico, including the Caribbean, the Bahamas, the West Indies, and Mexico. Some of the organisms are familiar, others not; some bite, some sting; others may be diseased or parasitized, which may make you wonder if they are edible; some contain poisons such as ciguatera, or high levels of pollutants such as heavy metals or pesticides, making them unsafe to eat.

We answer many questions by providing accurate and recent information about dangerous sea life and suggesting how to avoid getting stung or bitten; we offer means of safeguarding your health by proper preparation of your catch for eating; and include information on the effects of eating fish and shellfish from polluted waters.

If you are bitten, stung, or poisoned, the book provides first aid suggestions until you can get professional help. In all cases, if you are seriously injured, seek medical attention.

Some organisms are harmful to humans, either by nature or because of human-generated pollution. All marine creatures are subject to disease, infection, and infestation by parasites. When commercial fishermen, fish processors, and recreational fishermen find fish parasites or diseased fish, they generally want information about the parasite or disease and whether the fish is suitable for human consumption. Inquiries received at the University of Miami have come largely from sport and commercial fishermen, but physicians occasionally inquire what role marine parasites might play in human disease. Considerable information regarding poisonous fishes, fish parasites, and stinging and biting sea life and their roles in human health can be found in technical journals. However, those are not easily available to lay persons. In this book, we provide explanations which are easy to understand, and our directions are easy to follow.

Many cases of poisonous fish and shellfish have been reported from locations other than the east coast of the United States, the Gulf of Mexico, the West Indies, and the Bahamas. For some families of poisonous fishes in these waters, no valid records are available showing that they have caused human sickness or death; but since fishes in these families are poisonous elsewhere, they are presumed to be poisonous here, and are therefore included in this guide.

It is important to note that the mere lack of authentic records does not mean that a marine species or individuals of a species are safe to handle or eat, for the following reasons:

- The relationship between eating poisonous marine organisms and the illness is not always recognized.
- Identification of the sea life that caused the illness may be incorrect.
- Illness caused by marine animals frequently is not reported to health authorities.

Although this volume is written primarily for the east coast of the United States, the Gulf of Mexico, the Bahamas, and the West Indies, it has value elsewhere in other tropical and temperate marine waters where hazardous fish and shellfish occur. Common and scientific names may be different, but the avoidance and first aid principles may be very similar.

Some people scoff at the notion that certain marine animals are poisonous because, in their experience, they have never been troubled by these animals. This simply points out the normal variation in susceptibility and response of humans to poisons. Furthermore, a person's age or allergies may affect response to poisons. In this book, an animal is considered dangerous if any cases of poisoning, stinging, or biting have been authentically recorded.

The size and age of animals also can affect how dangerous they are to humans. For instance, regarding ciguatera, barracudas tend to be more poisonous when they are large, having accumulated more ciguatera toxin over the years. Similarly, shellfish exposed to human pollution for extended periods tend to accumulate more toxic chemicals and, when eaten, are more dangerous to humans.

Certain animals may be dangerous for more than one reason; for example, they may bite and their flesh may be poisonous to eat. The barracuda, shark, and moray fit this category; therefore, they are discussed under two or more chapters.

We selected photographs and drawings of the dangerous species that are commonly encountered in the region. In some instances, we also included photographs of closely related species for the benefit of our readers.

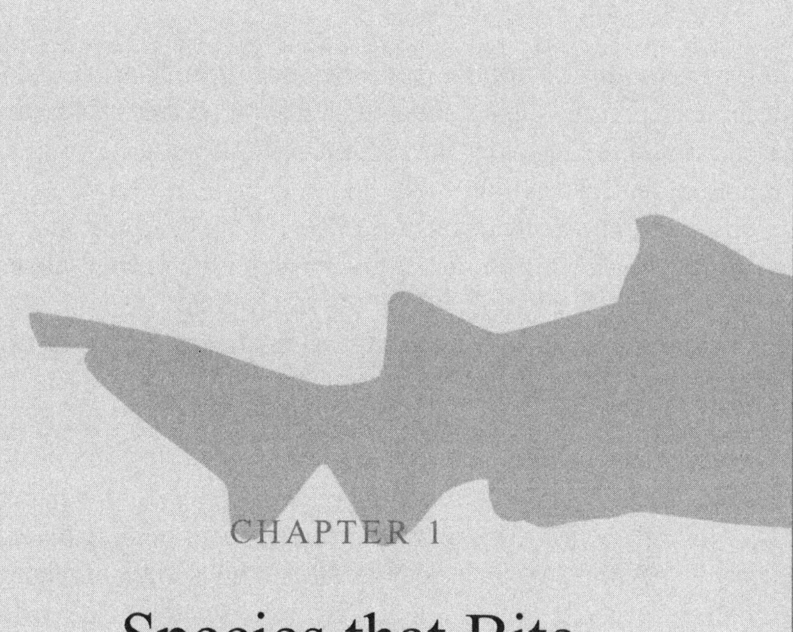

CHAPTER 1

Species that Bite

Many books are filled with information on "savage" marine animals, especially sharks. Recent popular books and films on shark attacks and the habits of sharks have greatly increased public awareness of the problem. In many beach resorts, considerable economic depression can result when shark attacks are sensationalized. A popular beach on Florida's east coast has averaged two shark attacks per year over the last twenty years, some of which have received nationwide attention in newspapers and on television. The accounts, written in a sensational manner, usually do not consider the number of swimmers using the beaches year-round. When viewed from the standpoint of numbers, one can see that the chance of being bitten by a shark is very small. Nonetheless, shark attacks are a very serious problem, especially if you happen to be a victim.

Sharks will not ordinarily attack humans, but like any large wild animal, their behavior is unpredictable and occasionally they can be very dangerous. Since they are powerful predators, it is best to stay out of the water when sharks are nearby. Comparatively few fatalities due to shark bites have been reported from Florida and Caribbean waters. However, by merely brushing against a swimmer, sharks can inflict serious wounds, caused by their sharp scales combined with the size and strength of the fish.

Considering the many aquatic activities of local people and tourists, one can say that unprovoked bite attacks on humans by other sea animals also are infrequent. Bites reported as caused by bluefish and barracuda are probably cases of mistaken identity by the fish. Since bluefish are voracious feeders that chase small prey fish along the beaches, swimmers occasionally get in their way and are bitten. Barracudas may see something flashing in murky water, such as a swimmer's jewelry, and mistake it for a prey fish with silvery scales. Moray bites occur when divers become curious or careless. A diver may not realize that a crevice into which he reaches may be occupied by a moray, which then bites in self-defense. Any animal, when cornered, is potentially dangerous. For first aid information, we refer to Additional Reading at the end of the chapter (Schimelpfenig and Lindsey, 1991).

How to avoid shark attacks and injuries

Numerous unsubstantiated stories exist about how to avoid injury from a shark attack. For instance, sharks do not always circle divers before attacking. Sharks are known to attack divers directly if they are provoked. Also, it is wrong to believe that you are safe from sharks if a school of porpoises is close by.

Many proven procedures for avoiding shark attacks are known. These include:

- Even if you are experienced, never dive or snorkel alone.
- Avoid the usual shark feeding times, i.e. early morning and evening.
- Do not wear shiny jewelry or brightly colored objects, since they attract sharks.
- Sharks are attracted by blood. A bleeding or wounded fish in a diver's net or on a spear will attract them, so get out of the water quickly. If a shark is very close, surrender your catch. Do not struggle with the shark over possession.

In discussing conditions accompanying shark attacks, Whitley (in Gilbert, 1963, page 342) stated that probably only a few species have made unprovoked attacks on humans in clear water that does not contain blood or refuse. But in turbulent or murky water, or under conditions in which there is bleeding from transporting a wounded, struggling fish, or where someone is attempting to net, spear, or otherwise capture a shark while in the water, many species of sharks are capable of inflicting injury to humans. Even the common nurse shark *(Ginglymostoma cirratum),* often considered harmless, will occasionally bite.

If a shark attack is imminent, probing or poking a shark's eyes or gills or even shouting under water or blowing bubbles may be an effective distraction. If these methods fail to scare it off, hit the shark with your fist, on the head if possible. Being alert, close to a boat, and with companions helps to avoid encounters with sharks.

See more on sharks, pp. 5–6.

How to avoid attacks from bony fishes

Barracuda: Avoid wearing shiny jewelry and carrying wounded or struggling fish in a dive bag or on a spear.

Bottom-dwelling species such as toadfish, angel shark, or flounder: Wear heavy footwear and shuffle your feet to avoid stepping on spines.

Reef-dwelling fish such as moray: Do not try to pull a moray from its hole. Do not reach into a hole or crevice for any reason.

Fish with strong teeth such as bluefish or seatrout: Use care in removing these fish from hooks. Bluefish will form schools when feeding on small prey fish in shallow water, get into a feeding frenzy, and bite waders. Avoid areas where fish schools are actively swimming and feeding. These areas can be noticed by disturbances in the water.

See more on bony fish, pp. 6–10.

How to avoid attacks from alligators and crocodiles

Keep a safe distance; do not walk close to the water's edge where these reptiles are known to live. They can hide under water and get up on land with amazing speed. Avoid investigating alligator and crocodile nests. The female alligator is usually close by and very aggressive about protecting her nest. The American crocodile is an endangered species and its nest and eggs must not be disturbed.

Do not feed alligators. This can cause them to lose their fear of humans and they could become very dangerous. In contrast, the American crocodile is much less aggressive and avoids humans.

Note that the American crocodile is a federally listed endangered species and protected by the Endangered Species Act.

See more on alligators and crocodiles, pp. 10–11.

Mollusks

Octopus *(Octopus* spp.)

Range: Tropical western Atlantic: Florida, Gulf of Mexico, Caribbean Sea, including north coast of South America.

Habitat: Rocky bottom, grassy areas.

Injury: The bite produces a small circular wound and welt; swelling, pain, nausea, headache, fever, and loss of appetite may occur.

Prevention: Do not handle an octopus.

Aid to Victim: Remove foreign material. Clean and disinfect the wound (see Chapter 2, "First aid for stingray wounds and other fresh wounds" p. 16).

Remarks: Reports of octopus bites are rare. *Octopus vulgaris* is a large and potentially dangerous species, whereas *O. joubini* is so small that it often occupies bivalve shells (Kaplan, 1982).

Color plate 1

Crustacea

Sea louse dermatitis isopod *(Rocinela signata)*

Range: Tropical western Atlantic: Florida Keys, Gulf of Mexico, Caribbean Sea, Central America, Cuba, Puerto Rico, St. Croix, and some of the Leeward Islands.

Habitat: Open coastal waters.

Injury: Isopods are small crustacean fish parasites (approximately 10 mm or 0.39 in), but may also accidentally attach to humans, causing painful bites inflicted by a biting apparatus that produces punctate hemorrhagic wounds. An anti-coagulant is apparently released by them. On rare occasions swimmers coming in contact with isopods are bitten. It appears that the isopods normally bite large specimens of fishes.

Prevention: According to divers in the Caribbean near the coast of Colombia, the greatest frequency of attacks by this species may happen during June to January in shallow (2 to 3 m or 6 to 9 feet deep), clear water with sea bottom covered by turtle grass *(Thalassia testudinum)* and scattered patches of fire coral *(Millepora alcicornis)*. If bites are occurring under those circumstances, leave these areas to avoid additional attacks.

Aid to Victim: Hydrogen peroxide can be used to clean the injured area and an antibiotic ointment applied to the wounds.

Remarks: Dr. P. Glynn, a coral reef researcher, states from personal experience that other species of isopods are known to bite humans.

Cartilaginous fishes (sharks)

Blacktip shark *(Carcharhinus limbatus)*

Range: Along the Atlantic coast from Massachusetts south to Brazil, including the Gulf of Mexico.

Habitat: Both offshore and nearshore waters. According to Robins et al. (1986), these sharks often come inshore in large schools, particularly in association with Spanish mackerel.

Injury: Although infrequent, shark attacks may occur in coastal waters. Bite wounds and lacerations can be serious and require immediate medical attention.

Prevention: Attacks can be avoided by staying out of the water when sharks are present. Avoid splashing while in the water. Do not carry speared fish next to your body.

Aid to Victim: Get medical attention as soon as possible. Control bleeding with pressure bandages until medical attention is available.

Remarks: The family Carcharhinidae (Requiem Sharks) includes a large number of sharks. Many of the genus *Carcharhinus* are difficult to identify to species. However, they are noted for their appearance as "typical sharks."

Color plate 23

> Local sharks
>
> Other possibly dangerous sharks in this geographic area include:
>
> Bull shark
> Blue shark
> Lemon shark
> Mako shark
> Reef shark
> Sand tiger shark
> Tiger shark
> White shark

Hammerhead shark *(Sphyrna zygaena)*

Range: From Maine to the West Indies.

Habitat: Inshore waters.

Injury: An attack by this shark may produce bite wounds or lacerations and the injury can be serious, even fatal. Sharks will often go into a feeding frenzy after inflicting an initial wound where blood is released.

Prevention: Leave the water when sharks are reported in the vicinity;

avoid splashing, do not carry speared or wounded fish on your person.

Aid to Victim: Get medical attention; antibiotics may be necessary. In case of large wounds, attempt to control bleeding with pressure bandages until medical attention is available.

Remarks: Comparatively few shark attacks occur considering the many swimmers, divers, and fishermen who use coastal waters. Some people have been bitten by usually sluggish nurse sharks after grabbing the tail or body of the fish. To be on the safe side, any large shark should be considered dangerous.

What to do if bitten by a shark

Numerous articles appear in the news media about swimmers' and divers' deaths caused by sharks; they often include photographs of the shark victims and illustrate the terrible wounds that the razor-sharp teeth can inflict, as well as the blood loss. However, experts point out that victims of the majority of bites survive if first aid is administered, beginning in the water. If not treated properly, even minor wounds can lead to serious infection. Most wounds, especially severe wounds causing considerable blood loss, require immediate medical attention. Shark bite victims may go into shock and they should be treated for that. Divers should be familiar with signs of shock, as well as first aid treatment, in order to treat their diving partner until medical help is available.

Bony fishes

Barracuda, great barracuda *(Sphyraena barracuda)*

Range: In the western Atlantic from Massachusetts to southeast Brazil.

Habitat: Inshore waters and on reefs.

Injury: Bite wounds, which can be severe. Pain and bleeding depend on the severity of injury. Wounds may be jagged.

Prevention: While diving, do not disturb large resting barracudas. Do not wear shiny, flashing objects while diving or snorkeling. Do not trail hands or feet overboard.

Aid to Victim: Clean and disinfect wounds. Get medical attention for large bites; antibiotics may be necessary.

Remarks: Most barracuda bites can be avoided by exercising care and avoiding behavior that will attract them, as in a case where a fisherman was bitten on the hand while rinsing off a dolphin fillet in the ocean.

Color plate 20

Bluefish *(Pomatomus saltatrix)*

Range: Nova Scotia and Bermuda to Argentina, but absent between southern Florida and northern South America.

Habitat: Bluefish generally school in large numbers along the east coast of Florida during March and early April and again in September.

Injury: Teeth are numerous, prominent, sharp, and compressed in a single series. Bluefish are voracious predatory fish. Their bites produce puncture wounds and lacerations. Pain and bleeding depend on severity of injury. There are many records of severe bites on the hands of fishermen.

Prevention: Leave the ocean when feeding schools of bluefish are moving along the beaches. Do not trail hands or feet from boat. Wear gloves and use caution when handling hooked bluefish.

Aid to Victim: Clean and disinfect wounds. Get medical attention; antibiotics may be needed.

Remarks: Along most beaches, lifeguards warn swimmers of approaching bluefish schools.

Color plate 31

Moray, spotted moray *(Gymnothorax moringa)*

Range: North Carolina and Bermuda, into the Gulf of Mexico southward to Brazil.

Habitat: Reefs and rocky bottom. Morays inhabit holes in coral or hide under rocks. Divers often see just the head of the moray projecting, while the body stays hidden.

Injury: The numerous large, sharp teeth are pointed inward to hold onto part of the body of a slippery prey, which is swallowed whole. Morays have poor eyesight and respond to odors and movements of possible food items. They almost never make an unprovoked attack on a diver; once they bite they tend to hold on for a short time. Bites result in puncture wounds, causing pain and bleeding.

Prevention: Generally divers are not in danger, especially if the moray sees the whole diver, not just an arm, fingers, or leg, which might be mistaken as one of their natural foods, such as a fish or an octopus. Morays locate their food mainly by smell. They can strike prey animals with remarkable speed. Avoid reaching into holes or into crevices looking for lobsters or other shellfish. Wear heavy gloves when diving and snorkeling.

Aid to Victim: If bitten, avoid pulling away from the moray. This will decrease the chance of tearing tendons and blood vessels. Stop the blood loss, and seek medical help as soon as possible. Clean and disinfect wounds. Mucus may cause infection of the wound. Obtain antibiotics if necessary.

Remarks: Long thought to be a very aggressive, vicious animal, the moray is now called gentle by some divers. Experienced divers and professional underwater photographers believe that neither description fits the moray. It should be regarded as any large wild animal with certain natural instincts and behavior patterns that may cause it to react unpredictably when a human invades its habitat.

Color plate 7

Sergeant major *(Abudefduf saxatilis)*

Range: Western Atlantic from Rhode Island south to Uruguay, including the northern Gulf of Mexico. Common on Caribbean reefs.

Habitat: Very common in shallow coastal waters and coral reefs, also found around floating seaweed (sargassum).

Injury: On reefs, sergeant majors behave similarly to the yellowtail snapper (described below). They may form large, rapidly swimming schools and occasionally nip and bite divers.

Prevention: Leave the area when feeding schools of sergeant majors are moving along the shallows or reefs.

Aid to Victim: Clean and disinfect any wound even if small. Get medical attention; antibiotics may be needed.

Remarks: Sergeant majors are small, highly territorial, and live up to their name. They "patrol" their area, usually a coral head, and chase intruders, whether fish, invertebrates, or snorkelers.

Seatrout, spotted seatrout *(Cynoscion nebulosus)*

Range: New York to southern Florida and entire Gulf of Mexico.

Habitat: Generally close to shore and in intertidal zones.

Injury: The upper jaw of this fish is armed with two large, pointed teeth, which can cause lacerations when fishermen handle it.

Prevention: Wear gloves and use caution when handling hooked spotted seatrout.

Aid to Victim: Clean and disinfect wounds. Get medical attention; antibiotics may be needed.

Remarks: This is a very popular recreational fish with good taste and lean flesh. When hooked the mouth is easily torn, hence the name "weakfish," of the related *C. regalis.*

Color plate 29

Flounder, summer flounder *(Paralichthys dentatus)*

Range: From Maine to Florida; most common north of Cape Cod.

Habitat: The summer flounder usually is found in summer in shallow depths near shore out to 120 feet, but it may occur down to 600 feet.

Injury: This fish has a large mouth with prominent, sharp canine teeth, which can cause wounds to fishermen when removing fish hooks.

Prevention: Wear heavy gloves and handle it with care.

Aid to Victim: Clean and disinfect wounds. Get medical attention; antibiotics may be needed.

Remarks: The species may reach a length of over 3 feet and a weight over 20 pounds. It is a popular and excellent food fish.

Toadfish, Gulf toadfish *(Opsanus beta)* **and oyster toadfish** *(Opsanus tau)*

Range: Western Atlantic from Maine to Cuba (oyster toadfish) and Florida, the Bahamas, and Gulf of Mexico (Gulf toadfish).

Habitat: Shallow waters over rocky bottom with rubble; also grassbeds and coastal bays.

Injury: Getting bitten by these fish may happen while wading or when a fisherman attempts to remove the fish from the hook. Toadfish have conical teeth and strong jaws, which can inflict wounds.

Prevention: Avoid touching the fish. Wear gloves or use fishing pliers. Wear shoes while wading in shallow water.

Aid to Victim: Clean and disinfect wounds. Get medical attention; antibiotics may be needed.

Remarks: Toadfish are camouflaged and lie still, often under rocks, which makes them difficult to see.

Snapper, yellowtail snapper *(Ocyurus chrysurus)*

Range: From Massachusetts southward, including Bermuda, to Brazil.

Habitat: Very common on shallow-water reefs of the Caribbean Region.

Injury: Yellowtail snappers swim rapidly in large schools, often over reefs and around divers, whom they occasionally nibble. They may reach a length of 2.5 feet and weigh about 5 pounds. When fish are being fed by divers, yellowtail snappers will occasionally gather in such large groups that they bite and peck humans in the water in the feeding excitement.

Prevention: Do not feed schools of snapper that are moving along the reefs.

Aid to Victim: Clean and disinfect wounds. Get medical attention; antibiotics may be needed.

Remarks: Yellowtail snappers are beautiful fish that add color and lively action to the reef community. See also Chapter 7: Human/Animal Interactions.

Reptiles

American alligator *(Alligator mississippiensis)*

Range: Southeastern coast of United States and the Gulf of Mexico. Relatively common in Louisiana and Florida.

Habitat: Mainly fresh water in tropical and subtropical wetlands. Alligators have also been observed in coastal marine waters.

Injury: Large jaws and teeth can cause massive bites. Alligators are very aggressive feeders. Adults have been reported to eat anything that moves and many things that do not, including rocks and human litter, such as plastic bottles. They can go for extended periods without eating and will gorge themselves when food is plentiful.

Prevention: Do not approach alligators. Above all, do not feed them. Avoid nesting areas. They frequently sun themselves along banks and can enter the water quickly and swim rapidly with their powerful laterally compressed tail, which they use to scull through the water. They also can run fast on land.

Aid to Victim: Attacks are usually extremely serious. Victims may be drowned or badly mutilated. If the victim is released by the alligator, medical attention is needed immediately.

Remarks: This large aquatic reptile may reach a length of 13 feet and weigh 600 pounds. It has a broad head, blunt snout, long body, and dark-colored thick skin. The eyes are located high on the head and the alligator is able to float low in the water, yet keep a sharp lookout for possible prey animals. The snout is rounded, not tapered as is the crocodile's, and the undershot jaws have strong, spiked, replaceable teeth. Natural food of young alligators consists of insects, small fish, and crustaceans. Although still a protected species, the alligator has made a comeback in recent years.

American crocodile *(Crocodylus acutus)*

Range: From southern Florida through numerous Caribbean Islands, Mexico, and Colombia.

Habitat: Fresh and brackish waters, saltwater bays, mangrove swamps, tidal wetlands in southernmost Florida.

Injury: No reports of crocodile attacks are known in south Florida. They are shy and usually not seen in populated areas. In other parts of the world, other species of crocodiles are known to attack humans when hungry. Their large teeth and powerful jaws can do serious injury or kill a person.

Prevention: As with alligators, do not approach crocodiles. Above all, do not attempt to feed them. Avoid nesting areas. They frequently sun themselves along banks and can enter the water quickly and swim rapidly with their powerful tail.

Aid to Victim: Although no attacks by American crocodiles are known, treatment would be the same as in case of alligator bites.

Remarks: Although similar to the alligator in overall appearance, the American crocodile can easily be identified by its narrow snout. Also, the strongly developed teeth of crocodiles are obvious even when their long jaws are closed. The crocodile is an endangered species in the United States. Of the approximately 20 species of crocodiles, the estuarine crocodile and the American crocodile are considered to be marine crocodiles. Known nesting sites of the latter exist in only a very few locations in extreme southern Florida. Most of these are in Everglades National Park, on northern Key Largo in the Florida Keys, and on the extreme south coast of the Florida mainland. They are monitored by the National Park Service, U.S. Fish and Wildlife Service, and Florida Fish and Wildlife Conservation Commission.

Color plate 27

Additional Reading

Avault, J. W., Jr. 1985. The Alligator Story. *Aquaculture Magazine* 11(4): 41-44.

Casey, J. G. 1964. Anglers' Guide to Sharks of the Northeastern United States, Maine to Chesapeake Bay. *Bureau of Sport Fisheries and Wildlife.* Circular No. 179: 32 pp.

de Sylva, D. P. 1963. *Systematics and Life History of the Great Barracuda (Sphyraena barracuda* Walbaum). Studies in Tropical Oceanography No. 1. University of Miami Press: 179 pp.

de Sylva, D. P. 1976. Attacks by Bluefish *(Pomatomus saltatrix)* on Humans in South Florida. *Copeia* 1976, No. 1: 196-198.

Fischer, W. (ed.) 1978. FAO Species Identification Sheets for Fishery Purposes, Western Central Atlantic. Fishing Area 31, Sharks, Vol. V. *Food and Agriculture Organization of the United Nations, Rome.*

Garzon-Ferreira, J. 1990. An Isopod, *Rocinela signata* (Crustacea: Isopoda: Aegidae), that Attacks Humans. *Bull. Mar. Sci.* 46(3): 813-815.

Gilbert, P. W. (ed) 1963. *Sharks and Survival.* D. C. Heath and Co., Boston: 578 pp.

Heemstra, P. C. 1965. A Field Key to the Florida Sharks. *State of Florida Board of Conservation.* Tech. Series 45: 11 pp.

Jackson, D. D. 1987. Alligators are Back, Breeding like Crazy and Making a Big Splash. *Smithsonian.* (January): 36-48.

Kaplan, E. H. 1982. *A Field Guide to Coral Reefs of the Caribbean and Florida, including Bermuda and the Bahamas.* Houghton Mifflin Company, Boston: 146-149.

Kensley, B. and M. Schotte 1989. *A Guide to the Marine Isopod Crustaceans of the Caribbaean.* Smithsonian Inst. Press, Washington, D.C.: 308 pp.

Lucy, J. 1980. Handle With Care. Mid-Atlantic Marine Animals That Demand Your Respect. *Sea Grant Program.* Virginia Institute of Marine Science. College of William and Mary, Gloucester Point, Virginia: 14 pp.

Menzies, R. J. and P. W. Glynn. 1968. *The Common Marine Isopod Crustacea of Puerto Rico. A Handbook for Marine Biologists.* Studies on the Fauna of Curaçao and Other Caribbean Islands. Vol. XXVII: 133 pp.

Randall, J. E. 1969. How Dangerous is the Moray Eel? *Australian Natural History.* (June): 177-182.

Ritchie, T. 1989. Marine crocodiles. *Sea Frontiers.* International Oceanographic Foundation. 35(4): 212-219.

Robins, C. R. et al. 1986. *A Field Guide to Atlantic Coast Fishes of North America*. Houghton Mifflin Co., New York: 354 pp.

Schimelpfenig, T. and Lindsey, L. 1991. *Wilderness First Aid. National Outdoor Leadership School*. NOLS Publications, Lander, Wyoming: 356 pp.

Schwartz, F. J. and G. H. Burgess. 1975. *Sharks of North Carolina and Adjacent Waters. Information series*. North Carolina Department of Natural and Economic Resources. Division of Marine Fisheries: 57 pp.

Seaman, W. Jr. (ed.) 1976. *Sharks and Man: A Perspective. Conference Proceedings. November 20-21*, 1975. Florida Sea Grant Report No. 10: 36 pp.

Webb, G. J. W., S. C. Manolis and P. J. Whitehead, eds. 1987. *Wildlife Management: Crocodiles and Alligators*. Chipping Norton, N.S.W. (Australia).

CHAPTER 2

Species that Sting

Everyone is familiar with stings by insects that cause great discomfort and, in extreme cases, can result in serious illness and even death. Some marine animals also sting, using structures that vary in size from tiny stinging cells in jellyfish to large spines on sea urchins, fishes, and rays. Toxic substances are discharged into the wound made by spines or stinging cells. Of the many venomous animals in the sea, only a few are harmful to humans. However, occasionally serious injury and even death has resulted from their stings. The Portuguese man-of-war *(Physalia physalis)* is virulent. At times, man-of-war and floating jellyfish become abundant and a problem to swimmers when onshore winds and currents carry them into shallow water and onto shores and beaches. Their long tentacles are often not seen by swimmers in the water or on the beach where they may be covered with sand or seaweed. When

Definitions

Sting: To prick or wound with a sharp point. Certain animals use a sharp, pointed organ to inject poison into a predator or prey organism.

Venomous organism: One having a poison gland or glands and able to inflict a poisonous wound by biting or stinging.

Venom: Poison secreted by some organisms.

venomous marine organisms die, they may still be dangerous for some time after death. Popular swimming beaches are routinely closed at times when Portuguese man-of-war are abundant.

Most people come in contact with a stinging marine organism accidentally, or they do not know it stings, or they do not see it. Accidental contact frequently happens with fire coral and fire sponge. They are brightly colored and often serve as hiding places for fish. On a number of local reefs, fire coral is one of the predominant structures, yet many people are not aware of this. Cone shells are searched out by shell collectors, but amateurs often do not know that the animal in the pretty shell can sting. Then there are the sea urchins and stingrays, which are often not noticed until the swimmer or wader steps on one.

How to avoid stings

When wading, swimming, or diving, some kind of foot protection should be worn, especially in areas where corals and sea urchins live. Avoid any animal with obvious spines, such as a sea urchin.

Shuffling the feet when wading gives a warning of your approach and gives the animal time to flee. It reduces the chance of stepping on a spiny or stinging animal, including those that may be partly or wholly buried.

Do not handle unfamiliar animals, especially fish with spines, jellyfish, or cone-shaped shells with a pattern design. Heavy gloves are recommended if you handle any of the species from these groups.

Avoid getting scratched by coral, since contamination causes infections and the wound may be slow to heal.

Although a fish may be dead, this does not eliminate the possibility of getting stung by venomous spines when handling it. Fishermen removing hooks from fish should exercise extreme caution.

First aid for stings by Hydrozoa and jellyfish

The principles of first aid are essentially the same for all stings by Hydrozoa and stinging jellyfish species. In severe cases, treatment should not be taken lightly, but considered an emergency requiring immediate medical attention. Fortunately, most jellyfish stings along the middle Atlantic coastal area are mild and superficial, and the recommended first aid consists of applying a dilute ammonia solution or vinegar to provide the victim with relief. There is a long list of popular first aid treatments, including unseasoned meat tenderizer, sodium bicarbonate, boric acid, lemon juice, tannic acid, canned milk, alcohol, and gasoline. In cases of mild stings a shift in pH will result and may give relief. For severe stings, treatments used by physicians and lifeguards should be followed. An important aspect of this treatment is to avoid using fresh water or hot water to rinse the wound, because this may discharge inactive stinging cells. This information is based on comments by Dr. F. E. Russell during a 1978 interview recorded in Lucy, J. (1980).

First aid for venom-injected wounds

Complete treatment for wounds that introduce venom into the victim's body includes many steps. Here we only mention basic first aid procedures.

Cleanse and flush a venomous puncture wound immediately. Urine is a nearly sterile fluid and can serve if no uncontaminated water is available. Heat the wounded area by immersion into hot water or use hot compresses to deactivate toxins. Poultices consisting of clean clay can also be used to counteract infections and remove toxic substances. Get medical attention; treatment for shock may be necessary. Drainage of the wound is important until any infection has healed.

First aid for stingray wounds and other fresh wounds

Because these types of wounds are often lacerations that may be followed by a secondary infection, it is wise to consult a physician. Large wounds may require sutures and antibiotic and anti-tetanus injections. As emergency treatment do the following: first wash the wound with uncontaminated water if available. Salt water is not recommended for washing because it may contain infectious bacteria, especially near shore. To clean and disinfect wounds, use compounds such as tincture of iodine or 70% alcohol. Remove any pieces of sheath or venom gland which may remain in the wound. These may look like shreds of grey mucus. Next, submerge the arm or leg in hot water, as hot as the victim can tolerate, for a period of 1/2 to 1 hour. Epsom salts may be added if available. Check again for foreign matter near or on the wound.

Hydrozoa

Fire coral *(Millepora* spp.)

Range: Tropical coastal waters in the western Atlantic.

Habitat: Coral reefs, also bridge and dock pilings and similar submerged structures.

Injury: Contact with fire coral produces welts, itching, pain, skin irritation.

Prevention: Wear gloves while diving or snorkeling on reefs. Avoid any contact with fire coral.

Aid to Victim: Apply alcohol or other antiseptic solutions.

Remarks: Fire coral is very common on many Florida reefs. It can best be recognized by its orange-yellow to mustard color and the arrangement of tiny pores in groups of six, a central larger one surrounded by five smaller ones.

Color plate 25

Man-of-war, Portuguese man-of-war *(Physalia physalis)*

Range: Throughout the world mostly in tropical waters. Those in the Atlantic spawn near the equator and southeasterly winds blow them along the east coast of the Atlantic Ocean from Florida as far north as Massachusetts.

Habitat: Open waters and coastal waters where large numbers occur in spring. Men-of-war's gas-filled floats drift on the ocean surface. Southeasterly winds will blow them onto beaches.

Injury: Contact with the tentacles, which contain venomous stinging organs, causes red welts on the skin, itching, pain, possibly fever, vomiting, paralysis. The tentacles may cling to the victim. Breathing may become difficult, the pulse rapid and feeble. A severe case may include unconsciousness. Get medical attention.

Prevention: Stay out of the ocean when warning signs are posted on the beaches. Stay a safe distance away from a man-of-war's gas float when swimming. Tentacles over 50 feet long have been reported. Do not disturb the Portuguese man-of-war on beaches, since the tentacles may spatter if the gas float bursts.

Aid to Victim: Remove all clinging tentacles from the victim's body with a towel or clothing. Apply alcohol or sun lotion to stop further action of stinging cells (nematocysts). External antihistamine creams and oral antihistamines help. Meat tenderizer is believed to be one of the best first aid remedies. Other external remedies include sugar, soap, vinegar, lemon juice, ammonia solution, sodium bicarbonate, boric acid solution, and papain. Also apply shaving cream and then shave the affected part with a safety razor. In severe cases, get medical attention.

Remarks: In case of a stinging, the Portuguese man-of-war is easy to identify by the large, gas-filled, blue-tinted float, which may reach 10 inches in length. Furthermore, when these organisms are pushed up on the beach by onshore waves there are numerous reports of stings by individuals walking along the beach. The stinging apparatus is quite large and is well described in scientific literature. Usually the largest invasion of Portuguese man-of-war in Florida occurs during spring. Warning signs are then posted along beaches. If a man-of-war washes ashore, do not step on the tentacles because even when dry they continue to sting for some time. Although often mistaken for a jellyfish (Class Scyphozoa) Portuguese man-of-war is actually a colonial organism of the Class Hydrozoa, and is related to fire coral.

Color plate 26

Scyphozoa

Jellyfish

Jellyfish (Class Scyphozoa, from the Greek words for "cup" and "animal") are generally rather large, about the size of a saucer. They are translucent with a variety of tints. Tentacles dangle from the margin of the body or "bell." Although they move with a pulsating motion to hold their position in the water column, for most species their major movement is determined by water currents. The jellyfish dangerous to humans have tiny stinging cells called nematocysts arranged on the tentacles. The structure and stimulation of nematocysts has been studied in detail. They contain a coiled thread with a barbed end. The thread is driven with some force, together with venom, into the prey animal (or person) that it touches. The size of the barb, the nature of the venom, and the victim's reaction to the stings vary between stinging species and severity of contact.

Dr. F. E. Russell (see note on First Aid above), an authority on the nature of venoms, points out that jellyfish toxins can be allergenic. A swimmer sensitive to the toxin can suffer anaphylactic shock from even a single stinging incident. It can result in muscle weakness, paleness, dizziness, possible tremors, and loss of consciousness, potentially leading to death. A nonsensitive person can become sensitive by repeated exposure to stings.

Thimble jellyfish *(Linuche unguiculata),* **seabather's eruption**

Range: Southern Florida, Cuba, Mexico, and the Caribbean.

Habitat: Shallow nearshore waters.

Injury: Contact with the larval stage of this species causes itching, usually under swimwear, while swimming in the ocean. Intense itching of the skin without eruption may last one week to ten days. Children are generally more likely than adults to have systemic symptoms. Redness, spotting, or other visible signs may appear on the skin.

Prevention: Unfortunately, at times when these organisms are abundant in the water, they are virtually impossible to avoid because of their tiny size. Therefore, when lifeguards or other swimmers report stinging organisms, it is best to stay out of the water until there is notice that the danger is past.

Aid to Victim: Shower thoroughly immediately after getting out of the water and rinse your bathing suit. Apply a hydrocortisone cream.

Remarks: The organisms are usually most abundant from May to September. The tiny, difficult-to-identify planula larvae have nematocysts (stinging cells) and drift away after making contact. Occasionally a welt, a red spot with a white margin, appears on the diver's skin. Tender areas of the body, such as the face, underarms, and areas under bathing apparel, are affected. It should not be confused with man-of-war stings.

Note: For many years, seabather's eruption was incorrectly referred to as "sea lice." However, "sea lice" are parasitic crustaceans (isopods) found in fresh and salt water, which infest fish (see Chapter 1).

Sea nettle or stinging nettle *(Chrysaora quinquecirrha)*

Range: From New England to Brazil.

Habitat: Most common in bays and estuaries in temperate and tropical seas.

Injury: In some areas sea nettles may occur in large numbers, making it difficult for swimmers to avoid them. After contact with a sea nettle's tentacles, the skin in the area of the sting turns red and swells, and a rash may develop. Severe stings can cause coughing, muscle cramps, and mucus discharge into the respiratory tract. A feeling of constriction of the chest may also result, inducing coughing, sneezing, and sweating.

Prevention: When these jellyfish float in the water column, sometimes in large numbers, get out of the water. Many more may appear in a short time. Avoid all contact.

Aid to Victim: Apply alcohol or solution of ammonia. Other remedies include vinegar, lemon juice, and soap. See "First aid for jellyfish stings," page 15.

Remarks: Fortunately, because of their large size (about 1 foot in diameter), sea nettles are quite visible and can usually be avoided.

Moon jelly *(Aurelia aurita)*

Range: Chesapeake Bay, Maryland and Virginia south to the Caribbean.

Habitat: Common on coral reefs. Drifting in the open sea and near shore.

Injury: In Chesapeake Bay stings by the moon jelly are quite mild; some reports state that they do not sting swimmers. However, in the Caribbean, the stings are clearly venomous. Contact produces itching, pain, localized redness and welts, and skin irritation.

Prevention: Upon seeing an individual moon jellyfish, get out of the water; many more may appear in a short time. Avoid all contact.

Aid to Victim: Apply alcohol or solution of ammonia. Other remedies include vinegar, lemon juice, and soap. See "First aid for jellyfish stings," page 15.

Remarks: Moon jellyfish are quite visible since they grow to a size of 1 foot in diameter, and can usually be avoided.

Lion's mane jellyfish *(Cyanea capillata)*

Range: Along the entire western Atlantic.

Habitat: Shallow coastal waters and estuaries.

Injury: The sting of this very large jellyfish with short tentacles is only mild. However, the effect of the sting may vary with the sensitivity of the person, and is more painful in the northern part of its range.

Prevention: Upon seeing individual jellyfish, get out of the water because many more may appear in a short time. Avoid all contact. Along the beaches, check with lifeguards regarding the presence of jellyfish.

Aid to Victim: Apply alcohol or solution of ammonia. Other remedies include vinegar, lemon juice, and soap. See "First aid for jellyfish stings," page 15.

Remarks: Lion's mane jellyfish are quite visible since they grow to a large size (may reach 6 feet in diameter), and therefore can usually be avoided.

Sea wasp or box jelly *(Chironex fleckeri)*

Range: Common in the Caribbean and occasionally found in southeast Florida.

Habitat: Coastal waters and the open sea.

Injury: The tentacles may reach 3 feet in length. Swimmers who come in contact with them may incur a severe rash that can cause excruciating pain.

Prevention: Upon seeing individual jellyfish, get out of the water since many more may appear in a short time. Avoid all contact. Along beaches, check with lifeguards about the presence of jellyfish.

Aid to Victim: Allergy medications might lessen the itching. White vinegar may do the same. See "First aid for jellyfish stings," page 15.

Remarks: There are several species of jellyfish in the genus *Chironex.* Some Pacific species occurring off the Australian coast are known to have killed swimmers.

Worms

Fire worm *(Hermodice carunculata)*

Range: Tropical waters.

Habitat: Reefs, inshore rubble.

Injury: Contact with the worm's bristles causes a burning sensation, swelling, numbness, and skin irritation.

Prevention: Avoid any contact with fire worms.

Aid to Victim: Remove bristles stuck in the victim's skin with tweezers, apply ammonia or alcohol.

Remarks: Usually found under rocks, this worm should not be handled without gloves.

Color plate 3

Mollusks

Cone shell *(Conus spurius* plus several subspecies, and *C. ermineus)*

Range: *C. spurius* extends from the Gulf of Mexico and Caribbean Sea south to Brazil. *C. ermineus* occurs in Florida and the Gulf of Mexico.

Habitat: Rubble bottom *(C. ermineus)* and sandy bottom *(C. spurius).*

Injury: Contact with the venomous stinging apparatus of a cone shell produces a puncture wound associated with immediate, sometimes intense pain on the site of injury, and later numbness. Tingling of the mouth area and extremities may develop, also tremor, nausea, vomiting, dizziness, and respiratory distress.

Prevention: Shell collectors should use heavy gloves. Avoid handling cone shells; it is especially dangerous to carry them close to your body.

Aid to Victim: Remove foreign material from the wound. Soak the area in hot water. In severe cases get medical attention.

Remarks: The venom apparatus of cone shells dangerous to humans is generally used by the animal to capture small fish. Not all cones are equally venomous. No record exists of poisoning from Florida or the Caribbean, but in other parts of the world fatalities or serious cases have been reported. Caution in handling cones is advised, especially if they are known to be capable of paralyzing or killing fish, as is *Conus ermineus.*

Sea urchins

Long-spined black urchin *(Diadema antillarum)*

Range: Florida and Bermuda to Surinam

Habitat: Rocky bottom, reefs, grass beds, pilings, sea walls. Shallow areas to 1,200 feet.

Injury: Stepping on or accidentally touching sea urchin spines may produce puncture wounds contaminated with sea urchin poison, causing immediate intense pain, localized swelling and redness, and in more severe cases nausea and respiratory difficulties. Spines broken off in a victim's skin can cause infection. They are brittle and difficult to remove. With time, they will dissolve in humans without harmful effects.

Prevention: Avoid all contact. Watch where you step while wading. Use footwear with heavy soles while wading in shallows.

Aid to Victim: If possible, remove spines and other foreign particles from wounds and use disinfectant such as alcohol or iodine. In serious cases get medical attention.

Remarks: Many sea urchins are not poisonous. However, since most have sharp spines, it is best to avoid any urchin encounter while wading. Eating gonads (eggs) of sea urchins may cause intoxication.

Color plate 21

Sharks and rays

Spiny dogfish *(Squalus acanthias)* **and Cuban dogfish** *(S. cubensis)*

Range: Spiny dogfish: Occurs in the western Atlantic from South

Carolina north to Labrador. Records also list the spiny dogfish in Florida waters. Cuban dogfish: Occurs along the western Atlantic coast of the United States from North Carolina, Florida, Cuba, Gulf of Mexico, and the Antilles south to Rio de Janeiro.

Habitat: Bottom-dwelling species, usually found from shallow water to 1,200 feet. Occasionally found near the surface where they have been caught by fishermen.

Injury: Directly in front of the two dorsal fins there is a strong, sharp, venomous spine. In order to defend itself, the fish will bend its body in the shape of a bow and strike at any object near it. Fishermen are often struck by the spines when they try to remove a dogfish from a hook, net, or spear. The puncture wound usually causes sharp intense pain occurring very soon after the spine is inserted, and may last for several hours, followed by general reddening of the skin and swelling.

Prevention: Wear heavy footwear when wading or on fishing vessels. When wading in areas where dogfish occur, always shuffle your feet, especially in waters that are murky. Wear heavy gloves when removing hooks from dogfish. Probably the wisest action is to simply cut the fishing line or leader.

Aid to Victim: Elevate the limb or body part where the wound is located. Bleeding should be facilitated and the wound irrigated, preferably with fresh water. Submerge the wounded area for at least a half hour at as high a temperature as the victim can tolerate. Get medical help.

Remarks: These sharks may reach a length of 4 feet. The chance of fishermen encountering spiny dogfish in the offshore waters of Florida or in the Bahamas is rather remote. With care in handling the dogfish the chance of harm is very low. Handling dead dogfish, as well as some other venomous fishes, requires considerable caution because the spine may still inject toxic venom.

Stingray, southern stingray *(Dasyatis americana)*

Range: New Jersey south to Brazil including the Gulf of Mexico.

Habitat: Grass beds and sandy bottom.

Injury: Contact with the venomous spine in the tail of the ray causes both lacerations and poisoning, as well as intense, rapidly spreading pain. Poisoning symptoms are mostly limited to the injured area. Possible symptoms include weakness, nausea, and anxiety. Less frequently observed are vomiting, diarrhea, sweating, and respiratory distress.

Prevention: Wear shoes while wading. Shuffle the feet on sandy bottom. Do not pick up stingrays.

Aid to Victim: Remove foreign material. Soak the wound in hot water for 30 to 90 minutes. Less severe wounds should be disinfected; however, severe lacerations need medical attention.

Remarks: Stingrays do not attack humans. The tail spine is used by the ray as a defensive weapon against predators. See "First aid for stingray wounds," page 16.

Color plate 34

Bony fishes

Scorpionfish *(Scorpaena* spp.)

Range: Scorpionfish belong to a large family of fishes, both in the Pacific and in the Atlantic. In the Atlantic they range from New England to Brazil, and the Gulf of Mexico.

Habitat: Coastal waters, including reefs.

Injury: The poisonous sting by dorsal, anal, and pelvic fin spines causes puncture wounds, pain, swelling, sometimes nausea, vomiting, headache, and diarrhea.

Prevention: Since many species of this genus can be found in shallow waters and grassbeds, use footwear while wading, and avoid contact. Fishermen should be careful when removing hooked scorpionfish from their gear.

Aid to Victim: Remove foreign material from the wound, soak in hot water, and disinfect. It may be necessary to get medical attention.

Remarks: Scorpionfish lie quietly in shallow water and are hard to notice because of their protective coloration.

Color plate 9

Catfish, gafftopsail catfish *(Bagre marinus)*

Range: Massachusetts south to Venezuela including the northern Gulf of Mexico. Present only in some areas of the West Indies.

Habitat: Inshore waters, including brackish waters.

Injury: Stings by pectoral or dorsal fin spines cause painful puncture wounds and swelling.

Prevention: To avoid the spines on fins when handling this fish, it is best to wear heavy gloves.

Aid to Victim: Remove all foreign material, as described above. Clean and disinfect all wounds.

Remarks: Fishermen may encounter these fish when angling or net fishing, and are injured by the sharp spines when removing them from a hook or a tangled net.

Color plate 33

Catfish, sea catfish *(Arius felis)*

Range: Massachusetts to south Florida into the northern Gulf of Mexico.

Habitat: Inshore waters, including brackish waters.

Injury: Stings by spiny rays on fins cause painful puncture wounds and swelling.

Prevention: Avoid the spines on fins. Handle with great care.

Aid to Victim: Remove all foreign material. Clean and disinfect wounds.

Remarks: This is a frequently caught catfish, but is not popular as a food fish. Sea catfish are considered a nuisance by anglers who find it difficult to remove them from hooks without being hurt by their sharp spines. Net fishermen have similar problems when the fish become entangled.

Cowfish, scrawled cowfish *(Lactophrys quadricornis)* **and trunkfish** *(L. trigonus)*

Range: Massachusetts and Bermuda to Central America and Brazil. Absent in the Gulf of Mexico.

Habitat: Reefs, inshore areas.

Injury: Handling these fish may cause puncture wounds, pain, bleeding, and swelling.

Prevention: Wear heavy gloves when snorkeling. Do not handle live cowfish.

Aid to Victim: Clean and disinfect wounds, as described above.

Remarks: Cowfish are unusually colorful fish that snorkelers and divers enjoy watching. Anglers and net fishermen should handle these fish with great care when removing them from fishing gear.

Color plate 5

Toadfish *(Opsanus* spp.)

Range: Western Atlantic from Maine to Cuba (oyster toadfish), and Florida, the Bahamas, and Gulf of Mexico (Gulf toadfish).

Habitat: Shallow waters over rocky bottom with rubble; also grassbeds and coastal bays.

Injury: These fish have sharp spines, and they can inflict a painful wound if given the chance (see also toadfish in Chapter 1, p. 9). Some tropical species of toadfish possess hollow spines attached to poison glands. However, these are not known to occur in our region.

Prevention: Avoid any contact.

Aid to Victim: Secondary infection can often occur with spine punctures. To reduce the chance, mild wounds should be thoroughly washed and bleeding encouraged to rid the wound of fish mucus and bacteria. For severe wounds, or if there is a broken fish spine imbedded in the wound, consult a physician. If, in the course of handling these fishes, slime or foam comes in contact with the eyes or other sensitive skin areas, rinse thoroughly and get medical attention.

Remarks: Toadfish are camouflaged and lie still, often under rocks. Swimmers and snorkelers in shallow water should be careful not to disturb the sea bottom.

Additional Reading

Abbott, R.T. 1974. *American Seashells.* Van Nostrand Reinhold, New York: 663 pp.

Arnold, R. E. 1973. *What to Do About Bites and Stings of Venomous Animals.* The Macmillan Co., New York: 122 pp.

Bücherl, W. and E. E. Buckley. 1971. *Venomous Animals and Their Venoms.* Vols. 2 and 3. Academic Press, New York: 687 and 560.

Dunn, F. D. 1982. Menacing Medusae, Horrible Hydroids, & Noxious Cnidarians. *Oceans.* 15(2): 6-23.

Edstrom, A. 1992. *Venomous and Poisonous Animals.* Krieger Publishing Co., Malabar, Florida: 210 pp.

Fischer, W. (ed.) 1978. FAO Species Identification Sheets for Fishery Purposes, Western Central Atlantic. Fishing Area 31, Vol. II. *Food and Agriculture Organization of the United Nations, Rome.*

Frankel, E. H. 1992. Seabather's Eruption Develops Following Mexican Vacation. *Clin. Cases Dermatol.* 4: 6-8.

Freudenthal, A. R. 1991. Seabather's Eruption: Range Extended Northward and a Causative Organism Identified. *Int. Oceanogr. Med. Rev.* 101: 137-147.

Halstead, B. W. 1980. *Dangerous Marine Animals*. Cornell Maritime Press, Centerville, MD: 208 pp.

Halstead, B. W. *Venomous Fishes*. In: Bücherl, W. and E. E.Buckley. 1971. *Venomous Animals and Their Venoms*, 2. Academic Press, New York: 587-626.

Hutton, R. F. 1952. Schistosome Cercariae as the Probable Cause of Seabather's Eruption. *Bull. Mar. Sci.* Gulf and Caribbean. 2(1): 346-359.

Hutton, R. F. 1960. Marine Dermatosis. *Arch. Dermatol.* 82: 951-960.

Lane, C. E. 1963. Man-of-War: The Deadly Fisher. *National Geographic* 123(3) 388-397.

Lucy, J. 1980. Handle With Care. Mid-Atlantic Marine Animals That Demand Your Respect. *Sea Grant Program.* VIMS. Educ. Series 26.

Moschella, S. L. 1951. Further Clinical Observations on Seabather's Eruption. *Arch. Dermatol.* 64: 55-56.

Osment, L. S. 1976. Update: Seabather's Eruption and Swimmer's Itch. *Cutis.* 18: 545-547.

Owre, H. B. 1956. Coelenterate Nematocysts as a Cause of Certain Kinds of Sea Stings. *Bull. Mar. Sci. of the Gulf and Caribbean.* 6(4): 309-314.

Russell, F. E. 1971. *Marine Toxins and Venomous and Poisonous Marine Animals.* Tropical Fish Hobbyist Publications, Inc., Neptune City: 176 pp.

Russell, F. E. 1980. Handle With Care. Mid-Atlantic Marine Animals That Demand Your Respect. *Sea Grant Program.* VIMS. Educ. Series 26.

Straus, J. S. 1956. Seabather's Eruption. *Arch. Dermatol.* 74: 293-295.

Tomchik, R. S., et al. 1993. Clinical Perspectives on Seabather's Eruption, also Known as Sea Lice. *Journal of the American Medical Association.* 269: 1660-1672.

Wong, D. E., et al. 1994. Seabather's Eruption. Clinical, Histologic, and Immunologic Features. *Journal of the American Academy of Dermatology.* 30 (3): 399-406.

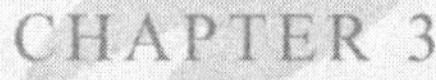

CHAPTER 3

Species Dangerous to Eat

Types of poisons in fish and shellfish

The most frequent types of poisoning associated with eating fish are ciguatera, scombroid, and puffer poisoning. Because of frequent incidents, some general precautions follow below. Note that the poisons mentioned above should not be confused with ptomaine poison, produced in a variety of foods by spoilage, nor with allergic reactions and shellfish poisons.

Eating seafood

Seafood is gaining in popularity in North America, due in a large part to its lower cholesterol levels compared to red meat. High cholesterol levels are said to be a cause of the increase in heart attacks over the past decades. American Heart Association studies show that diets relying mainly on fish result in fewer coronary attacks in middle-aged men. Interestingly, this is based on the beneficial effect of unsaturated oils present in seafoods. Aside from their low saturated fat content, they supply in balanced amounts the valuable amino acids needed by humans, and have been heralded for their high content of certain essential minerals and water-soluble vitamins.

Before eating unfamiliar fish, consider the following:

- If fish are obtained from an unfamiliar area, seek local advice about their edibility. Some areas in the Caribbean are notorious for a variety of ciguatoxic fish.
- Avoid eating large specimens, especially barracudas, snappers, jacks, and groupers. Fish with "beaks," such as parrotfish, eat algae and should be avoided since they may accumulate poisons.
- Avoid eating fish taken from waters polluted, or suspected of being polluted, by human waste, such as waters near sewage outfalls.
- Do not eat fish that expand when captured or disturbed, such as puffers and porcupinefish (color plate 22). Do not eat fish that have no visible scales, like puffers.
- Fish skin, head, and internal organs, especially the liver and gonads, should not be consumed.
- If the flesh has a decided "off flavor" or stings the mouth, discard it.

Shellfish poisons

Filter-feeding mollusks may accumulate toxins from some species of phytoplankton, which may cause serious illness when eaten. Paralytic shellfish poisoning, also called mussel or clam poisoning, paresthetic poisoning, or mytilitoxification poisoning, is caused by eating shellfish that have been feeding on certain species of toxic dinoflagellates. Other diseases caused by eating toxic shellfish are called, variously, neurotoxic shellfish poisoning (NSP), diarrhetic shellfish poisoning (DSP), and amnestic shellfish poisoning (ASP), all caused by shellfish that consume toxic phytoplankton.

First aid for eating toxic fish or shellfish

The many symptoms produced by different toxins show considerable similarity. Unfortunately, both diagnosis and treatment are difficult and nearly always require medical attention.

For emergency first aid, cause vomiting to empty the patient's stomach as soon as possible. Small amounts of charcoal or chalk administered internally in powdered form may absorb the toxin if medical help is not readily available. After the stomach has been completely emptied, considerable amounts of liquid should be taken, and the victim needs to rest.

Human allergies to seafood

Allergies are the result of a response by the body's immune system to invasive agents perceived to be dangerous to the body. The mechanism of the body's response is rather complicated and will not be discussed here. Some people have an allergy to fish and shellfish, manifested by stomach or intestinal disorders (nausea, vomiting), hives, or swelling of the eyes, lips, face, tongue, and throat. Some cases may lead to an anaphylactic reaction, including narrowing of air passageways, rapid pulse, a drop in blood pressure, cardiovascular collapse, and shock, a life-threatening condition. This requires immediate medical attention.

Tracking the substances that cause allergic responses can be involved and costly. However, if the response to eating a certain kind of seafood is rapid, the victim should simply avoid that type of seafood, especially if the response to it occurs more than once.

Species affected by natural events

In addition to parasites, there are many diseases of fish and shellfish that result from natural causes. They may be indirectly affected by human-generated domestic, industrial, and agricultural pollution. Natural causes, such as acute temperature changes, decomposition of organic matter, lack of oxygen, and poisons released by tiny marine organisms (such as red tide caused by toxic plankton, Kudo, 1971), may be hard to pinpoint. Fish diseased or distressed by natural causes often appear in large numbers and are usually accompanied by dead or dying fish. In cases of mass mortalities, such conditions affect not only many fish, but frequently fish of a wide variety of species, as in the case of red tides, which kill species of both invertebrates and vertebrates. Since the cause of disease or distress is often not known or is difficult to determine, it is advisable not to eat fish behaving unnaturally, or any caught in the vicinity of dead or dying fish.

Spoiled seafood

Seafood is probably the most perishable of all foods and is particularly susceptible to spoilage by bacteria, autolysis-enzymatic action, and oxidation-rancidity of fatty acids. The most important groups of bacteria which cause spoilage of seafood and sickness in humans are *Pseudomonas* spp., *Salmonella* spp., and *Achromobacter* spp. Iced fish can have all three groups present because these bacteria survive and grow near freezing level (20 to 32° F).

Regarding enzymatic spoilage, a protein produced by fish functions as a catalyst in living organisms. The action does not stop upon death of the fish, and flavor, tissue color, and texture of the flesh are changed. In herring, the color change caused by this process is called "rusting."

The process is indicated by oxidation, resulting in a varnishlike odor. Oily fish, such as herring, mackerel, and salmon, are more subject to oxidation than other fish.

How to tell if fish are fresh

Fresh fish can be identified by a firm, elastic feel of the flesh; belly not bulging; no "fishy" odor; eyes bright, transparent, and not shrunken; gills bright red; and skin not faded. Of all the tests of fresh fish and shellfish, smell is one of the best. Also, shrimp held on ice for extended periods develop black spotting. To improve the appearance of the shrimp for market, the spots can be removed by a sodium bisulfite dip, approved by the U.S. Food and Drug Administration (FDA), which has standards on residue of this chemical in the shrimp flesh. Concentrated sodium bisulfite dips can leave an undesirable "off" taste. Good handling practices start aboard the vessel and should not wait until fish reach the processing plant.

Bacteria: Cholera

Cholera is caused by a bacterial pathogen, *Vibrio cholerae*, which has produced epidemics in human populations well back in mankind's recorded history. Today, it flares up in areas of the world where the poor live without sewage treatment, come in contact with contaminated drinking water, and eat fruits and vegetables grown in fields irrigated with untreated water. In these same communities, people may eat raw fish and shellfish washed with contaminated water, thereby spreading the disease. Usually within a few hours after infection, the victim shows symptoms such as vomiting, acute diarrhea, and extreme dehydration. Death is caused by shock, kidney collapse, and circulatory arrest. The death rate from cholera is very high. The 1991 outbreak of cholera, which was traced to Lima, Peru, spread rapidly from southern Mexico south to Argentina, affecting approximately 70,000 people along a 1,200-mile coast line. During 1991 an estimated 1,000 or more Peruvians died from cholera. The Peruvian fish export business came to a halt. In contrast, up-to-date treatment of sewage and drinking water and better regulated fish processing plants resulted in fewer cases of cholera in North America.

Raw oysters and bacteria

American oyster *(Crassostrea virginica)*

Range: On the Atlantic Coast of North America from the Canadian Maritimes southward around Florida, and all along the Gulf of Mexico to the West Indies and Venezuela.

Habitat: Mangroves, flats, inshore banks.

Injury: Persons with chronic illnesses of the liver, stomach, or blood, or who suffer from immune disorders, cancer, alcoholism, diabetes, or AIDS, are at a greater risk of serious illness or death from raw oysters. The causative agent is a bacterium, *Vibrio vulnificus*, which occurs naturally in marine waters, especially warm tropical and subtropical waters. From 1981 to 1995, over 100 people were infected with *V. vulnificus* and 48 died. There are believed to be over 100 types or strains of this bacterium. The infection can grow rapidly throughout the human body. Within 12 to 24 hours after contact with the bacterium, symptoms such as chills, leg pain, vomiting, and diarrhea begin, and persist as the infection spreads.

Prevention: If a person has any of the chronic illnesses listed above, it is advisable to consult a physician before eating raw or lightly cooked oysters. It is best to eat oysters that are fully cooked. Note also that most infections occur during spring months.

Aid to Victim: Medical treatment, which includes high doses of antibiotics.

Remarks: Healthy consumers usually do not need to worry about this type of infection.

Paralytic shellfish poisoning (PSP)

American oyster *(Crassostrea virginica)*

Range: On the Atlantic Coast of North America from the Canadian Maritimes southward around Florida, and all along the Gulf of Mexico to the West Indies and Venezuela.

Habitat: Mangroves, flats, inshore banks.

Injury: Paralytic shellfish poisoning, caused by biotoxins accumulated in oysters. Symptoms include tingling of lips, tongue, and face, which may turn to numbness, constrictive sensation in the throat, and incoherent speech. Dizziness, headache, weakness, perspiration, respiratory, distress, and paralysis may occur (Sindermann, 1990).

Prevention: Avoid eating shellfish from areas where known cases of this poisoning are being reported. Obtain up-to-date information from local health authorities.

Aid to Victim: No specific antidote is known. Treatment is largely symptomatic. Get medical attention.

Remarks: The quality of oysters on fishing grounds can change rather rapidly, hence it is advisable to inquire frequently. According to a recent study by a University of Alaska scientist, dinoflagellates and marine bacteria may combine to produce the toxins that cause paralytic shellfish poisoning. Contrary to some beliefs, no cooking procedures will destroy these toxins.

Rock crab *(Cancer irroratus)*

Range: From Labrador south to the eastern coast of Florida.

Habitat: Cold water species ranging in depth from the low water mark to 1,800 feet.

Injury: Paralytic shellfish poisoning. Toxins may accumulate in larger decapods, such as crabs, lobsters, etc., as a result of their ingestion of toxic food sources. Since the rock crab feeds mainly on sea urchins and other invertebrates, which in turn feed on microscopic plankton (predominantly dinoflagellates), the rock crab may be a secondary transvector. Symptoms include tingling of lips, tongue, and face, which may turn to numbness; constrictive sensation in the throat; and incoherent speech. Dizziness, headache, weakness, perspiration, respiratory, distress, and paralysis may occur.

Prevention: Do not eat rock crabs from areas declared unsafe by government authorities.

Monitoring and surveillance systems of crabs are necessary to avoid paralytic shellfish poisoning in consumers.

Aid to Victim: Get medical attention in severe cases.

Remarks: Public health authorities can provide information on safety of local crab beds.

Interestingly, the American lobster *(Homarus americanus)* does not accumulate the poison in spite of a diet similar to the rock crab.

Surf clam *(Spisula solidissima)*

Range: Along the eastern coast of North America, from Nova Scotia to South Carolina.

Habitat: Open ocean below the low water line down to 100 feet, on sandy bottom.

Injury: Paralytic shellfish poisoning. Biotoxins accumulated by surf clams. Symptoms include tingling of lips, tongue, and face which may turn to numbness, constrictive sensation in the throat, and incoherent speech. Dizziness, headache, weakness, perspiration, respiratory distress, and paralysis may occur.

Prevention: Do not eat clams from areas declared unsafe by government authorities.

Aid to Victim: Get medical attention in severe cases.

Remarks: Public health authorities can provide information on safety of local clam beds.

Bay scallop *(Argopecten irradians)*

Range: Atlantic Coast of the United States, from Massachusetts southward to the Caribbean Sea, including Colombia.

Habitat: Nearshore and estuarine waters.

Injury: Paralytic shellfish poisoning. Scallops feed by filtering algae and diatoms, protozoa and detritus. Biotoxins may accumulate. Symptoms include tingling of lips, tongue, and face which may turn to numbness, constrictive sensation in the throat, and incoherent speech. Dizziness, headache, weakness, perspiration, respiratory distress, and paralysis may occur.

Prevention: Do not eat scallops from areas declared unsafe by government authorities.

Aid to Victim: Get medical attention in severe cases.

Remarks: Public health authorities can provide information on safety of local scallop beds.

Sea scallop *(Placopecten magellanicus)*

Range: Labrador to Cape Hatteras, North Carolina.

Habitat: In the northern part of their range, sea scallops occur in shallow water of less than 60 feet, while in the southern part they are found in much deeper water, beyond 180 feet.

Injury: Paralytic shellfish poisoning. Scallops feed by filtering algae and diatoms, protozoa and detritus, although occasionally crustaceans, polychaetes, echinoderms, and seaweeds are found in their stomachs.

Biotoxins may accumulate. Symptoms include tingling of lips, tongue, and face which may turn to numbness, constrictive sensation in the throat, and incoherent speech. Dizziness, headache, weakness, perspiration, respiratory distress, and paralysis may occur.

Prevention: Do not eat scallops from areas declared unsafe by government authorities.

Aid to Victim: Get medical attention in severe cases.

Remarks: Public health authorities can provide information on safety of local scallop beds.

Neurotoxic poisoning (NP)

Red tide *(Ptychodiscus brevis*, **formerly** *Gymnodinium breve)*

Range: Along the coast of Florida and the southern coast of Texas, extending down the coast of Mexico and Trinidad, including the Orinoco River in the Gulf of Paria, Venezuela (the latter not well documented).

Habitat: Warm coastal waters.

Injury: Red tide, caused by single-cell organisms (dinoflagellates) that live free in the water, is responsible for the loss of valuable fish and shellfish. When conditions are suitable, these protozoa suddenly reproduce in great numbers, causing a "bloom." The toxin they produce kills a wide variety of marine organisms. In humans, symptoms are respiratory irritation from breathing aerosols of the red tide, and irritation of the skin of swimmers.

Prevention: Find out from the local health authority if it is safe to eat fish and shellfish from areas of a bloom. Avoid inhaling toxic red tide air. Leave the water at the first sign of skin irritation from red tide, and leave the affected area if possible.

Aid to Victim: Move the victim from the immediate vicinity of the red tide occurrence.

Remarks: It is still not clearly understood what causes red tide blooms to occur in one year and not another. Although there have been many reports of "red tides," only recently has the responsible organism been identified. Early reports were based on the color of the water and the appearance of dead fish.

Diarrhetic shellfish poisoning (DSP)

Soft clam, soft-shell clam, also called longneck and steamer clam *(Mya arenaria)*

Range: From Labrador to North Carolina, coastal waters.

Habitat: After passing through larval stages, the clams metamorphose and settle to the bottom, moving short distances, and as they get older they dig a permanent burrow and remain there.

Injury: Diarrhetic shellfish poisoning. Symptoms include cramps; severe diarrhea; nausea, vomiting, and chills. Death is rare. Two species of dinoflagellates are the cause.

Prevention: Do not eat soft clams from areas declared unsafe by government authorities.

Aid to Victim: Get medical attention in severe cases.

Remarks: The dinoflagellates may poison several different species of bivalves.

Amnestic shellfish poisoning (ASP), domoic acid

Blue mussel *(Mytilus edulis)*

Range: In the western Atlantic from lower Arctic Ocean south to South Carolina.

Habitat: The blue mussel attaches by a multi-threaded byssus spun by a short foot, usually to floating logs, dock pilings, and intertidal rocks.

Injury: In 1987, an outbreak of amnestic shellfish poisoning in mussels from the vicinity of Prince Edward Island, Canada, poisoned an estimated 150 people. Twenty-two were hospitalized, ten required intensive care, and two died. Among the neurologic responses are memory loss and disorientation and, in severe cases, death. The causative agent is believed to be a diatom.

Prevention: Do not eat mussels from areas declared unsafe by government authorities.

Aid to Victim: Get medical attention in severe cases.

Remarks: Public health authorities can provide information on safety of local mussel beds. Amnestic shellfish poisoning symptoms from Sindermann (1990) are the following: nausea, vomiting, muscle weakness, disorientation, and loss of short-term memory.

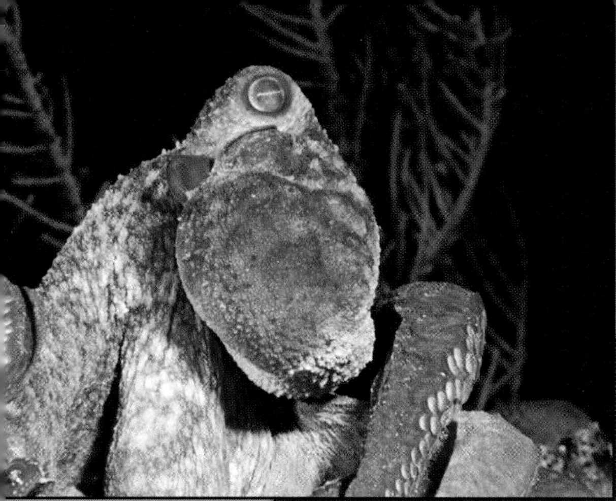

1. *Octopus* sp.
page 4

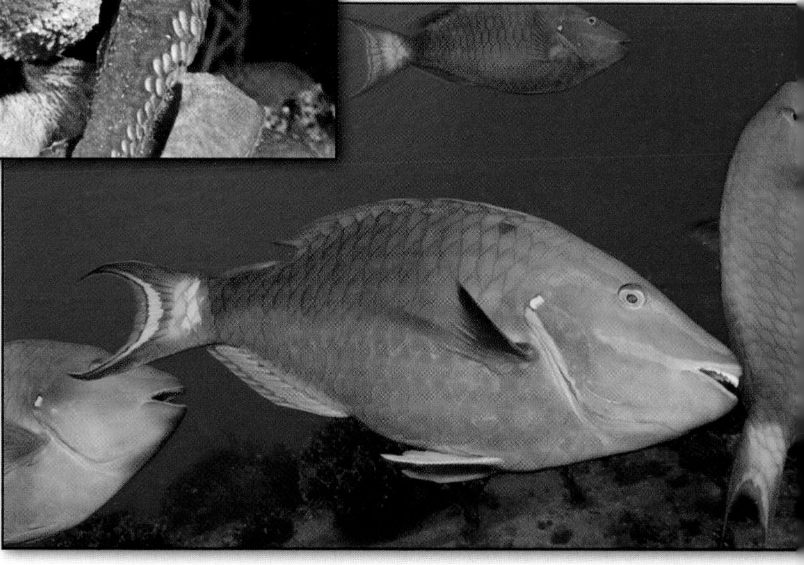

2. Stoplight Parrotfish
(Sparisoma viride)
page 41

3. Fire Worm
(Hermodice carunculata)
page 21

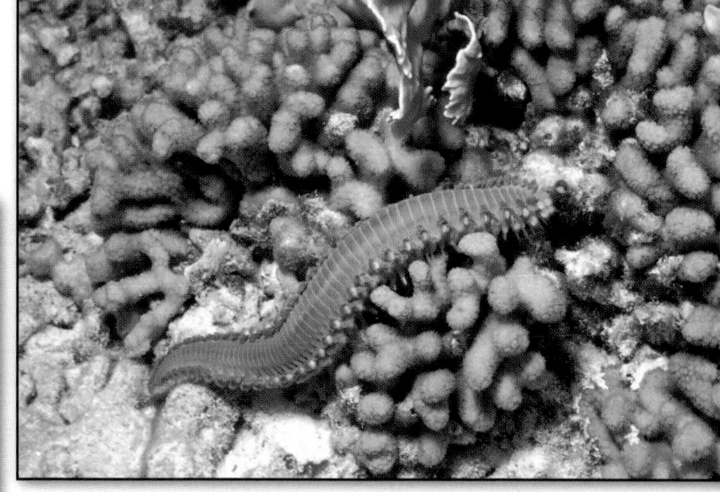

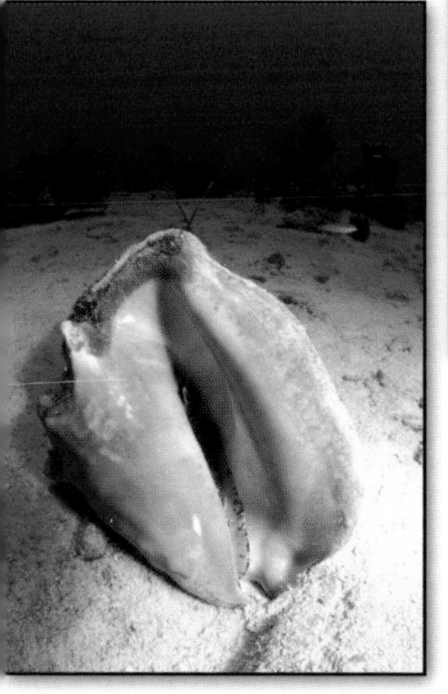

4. Queen Conch *(Strombus gigas)*
page 37

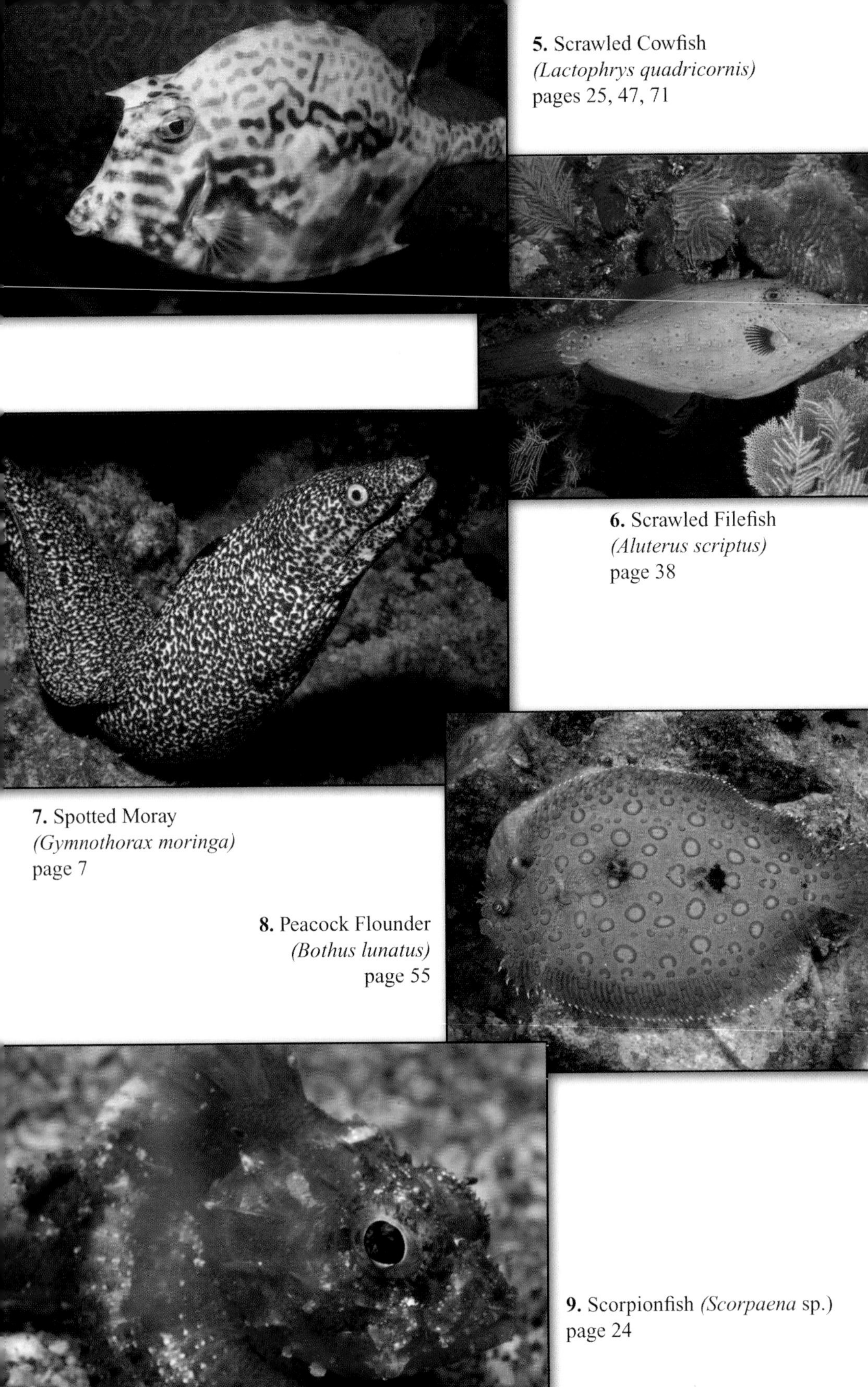

5. Scrawled Cowfish
(Lactophrys quadricornis)
pages 25, 47, 71

6. Scrawled Filefish
(Aluterus scriptus)
page 38

7. Spotted Moray
(Gymnothorax moringa)
page 7

8. Peacock Flounder
(Bothus lunatus)
page 55

9. Scorpionfish *(Scorpaena* sp.)
page 24

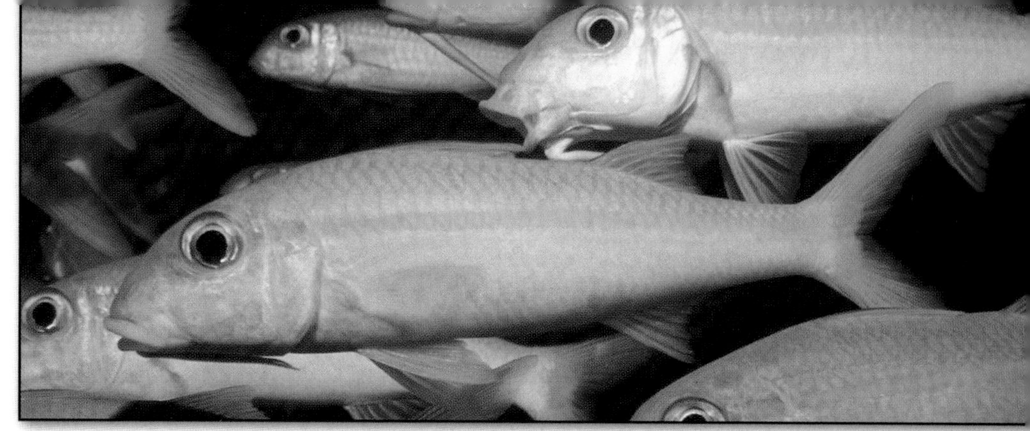

10. Yellow Goatfish *(Mulloidichthys martinicus)* page 39

11. High Hat *(Equetus acuminatus)* page 55

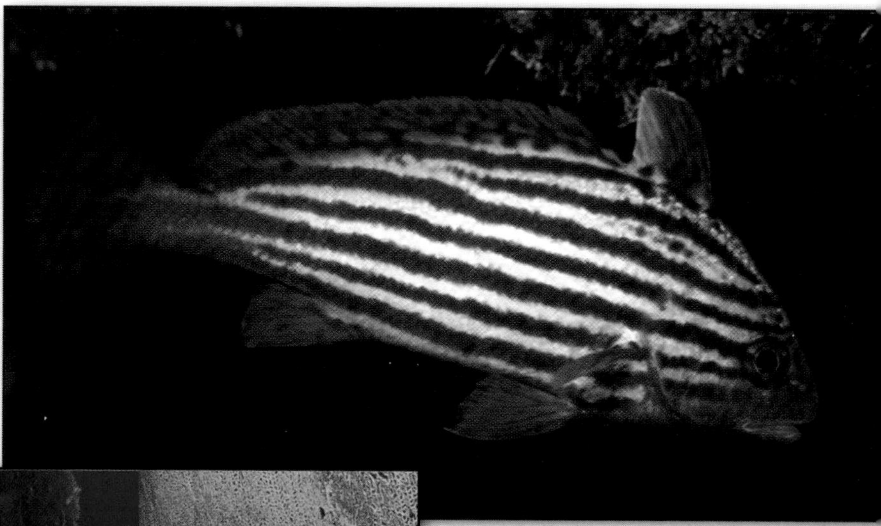

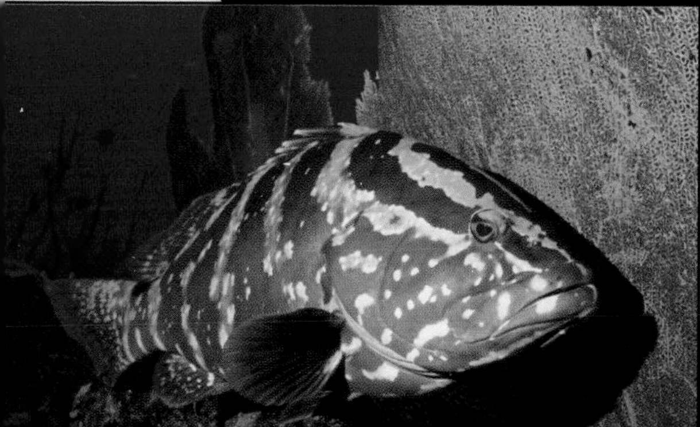

12. Nassau Grouper *(Epinephelus striatus)* pages 43, 56

13. Hogfish *(Lachnolaimus maximus)* page 39

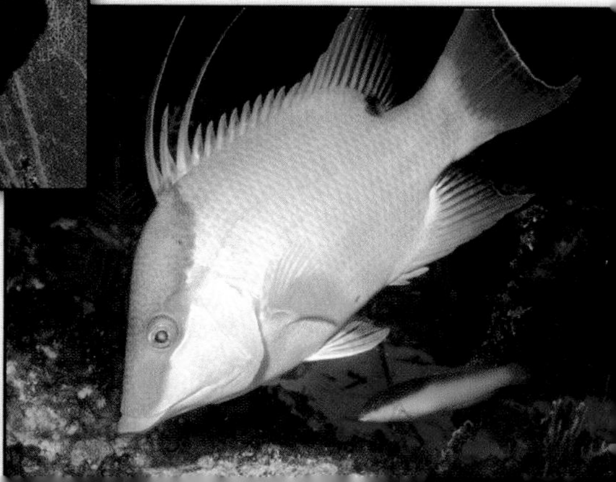

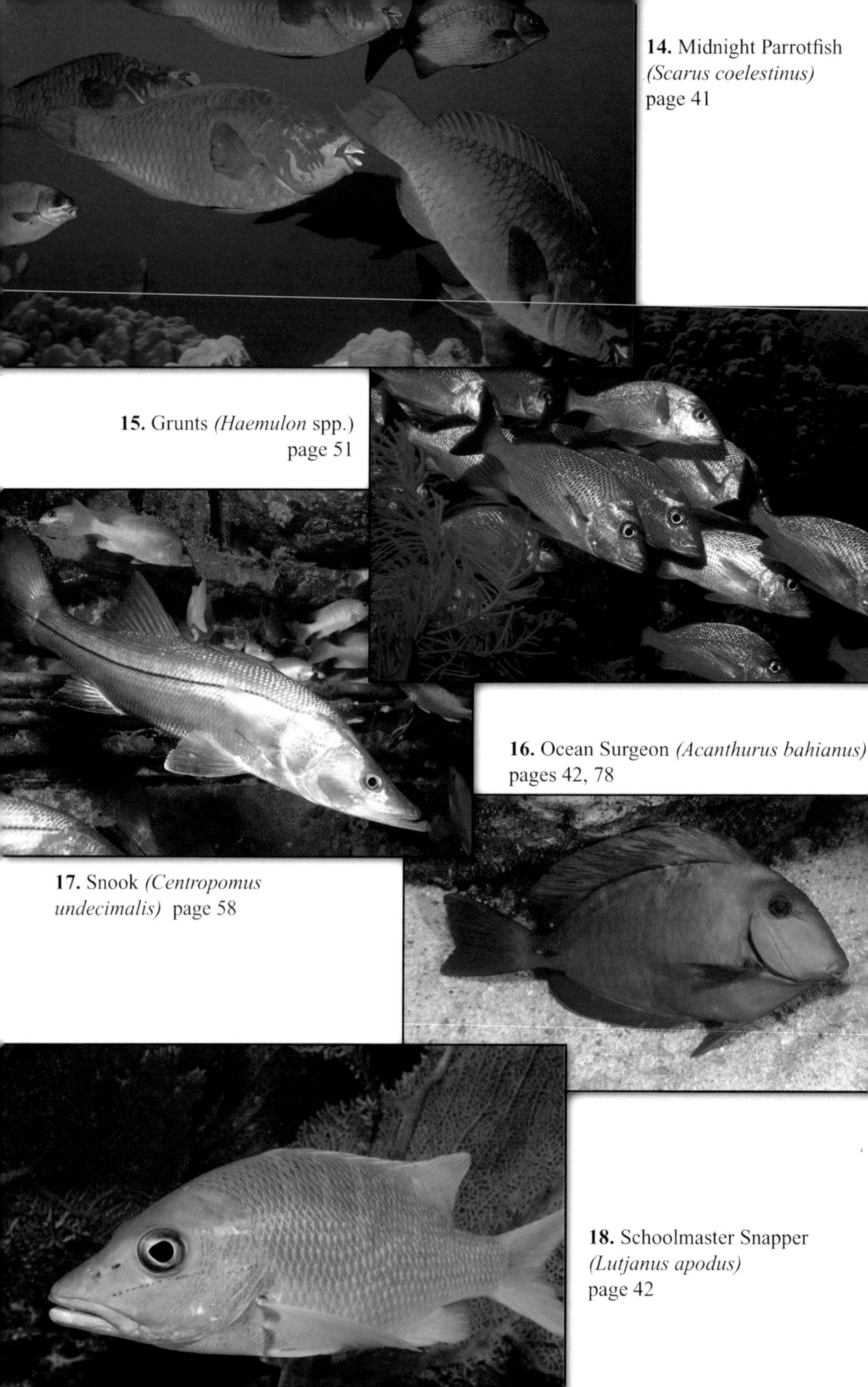

14. Midnight Parrotfish *(Scarus coelestinus)* page 41

15. Grunts *(Haemulon* spp.) page 51

16. Ocean Surgeon *(Acanthurus bahianus)* pages 42, 78

17. Snook *(Centropomus undecimalis)* page 58

18. Schoolmaster Snapper *(Lutjanus apodus)* page 42

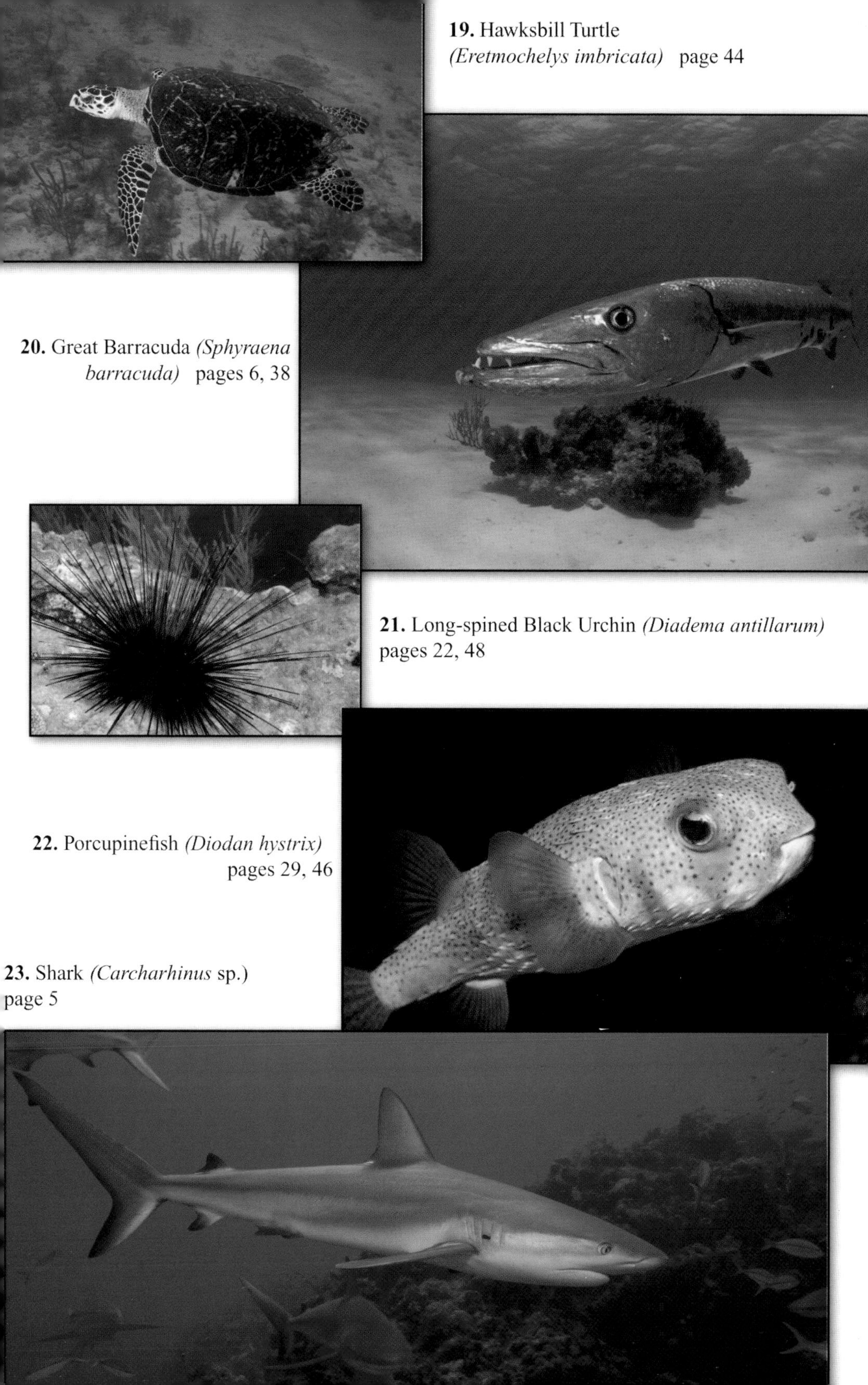

19. Hawksbill Turtle
(Eretmochelys imbricata) page 44

20. Great Barracuda *(Sphyraena barracuda)* pages 6, 38

21. Long-spined Black Urchin *(Diadema antillarum)* pages 22, 48

22. Porcupinefish *(Diodan hystrix)* pages 29, 46

23. Shark *(Carcharhinus* sp.) page 5

24. Blue Crab *(Callinectes sapidus)* page 59

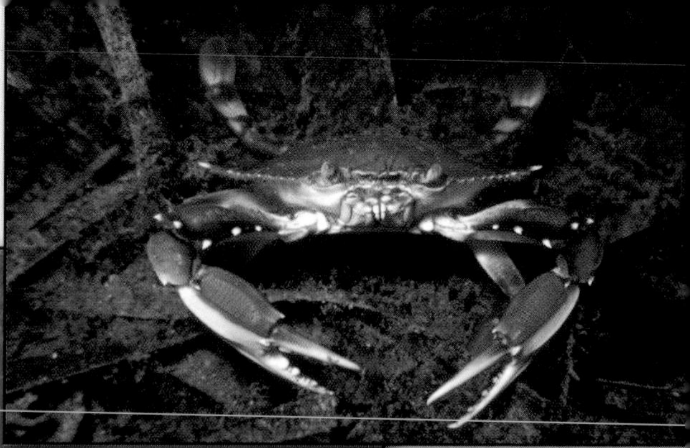

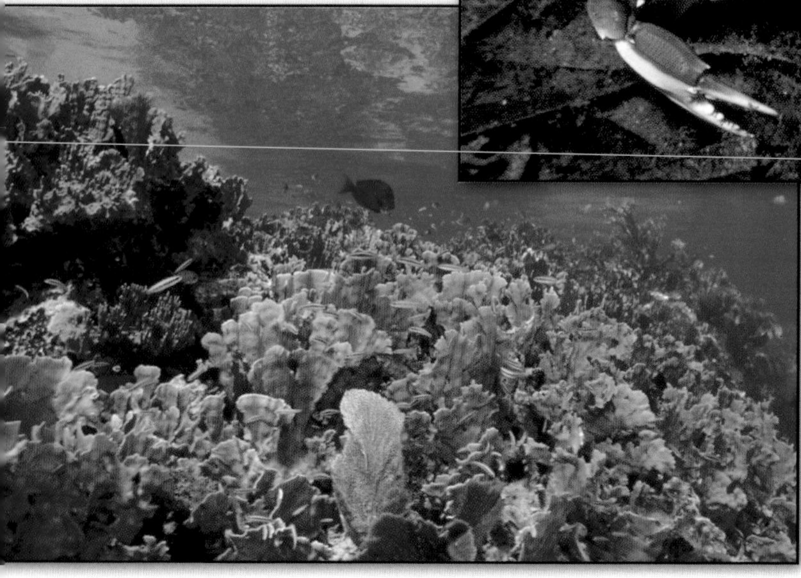

25. Fire Coral *(Millepora* sp.) page 17

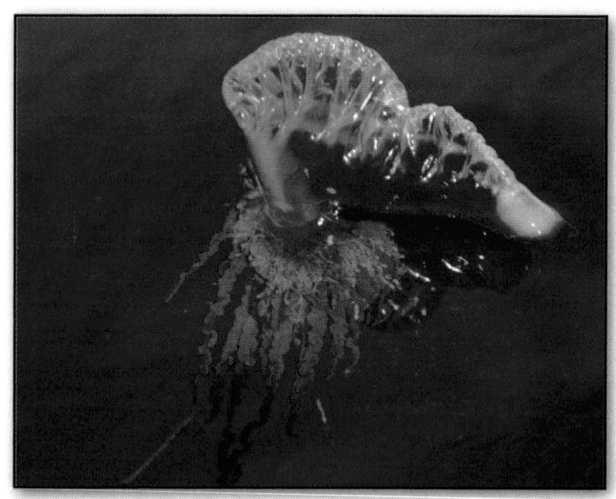

26. Portuguese Man-of-War *(Physalia physalis)* page 17

27. American Crocodile *(Crocodylus acutus)* page 11

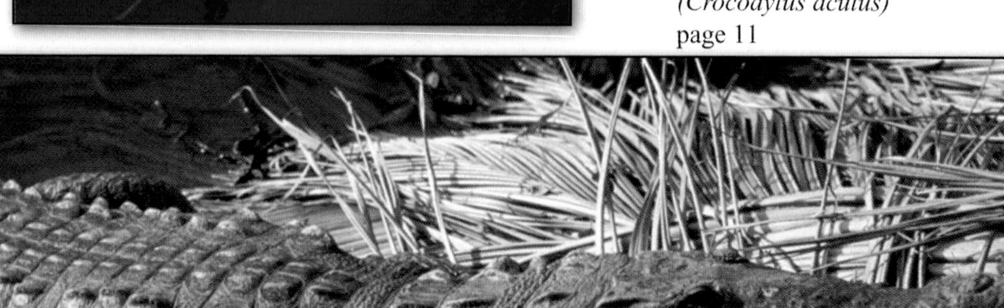

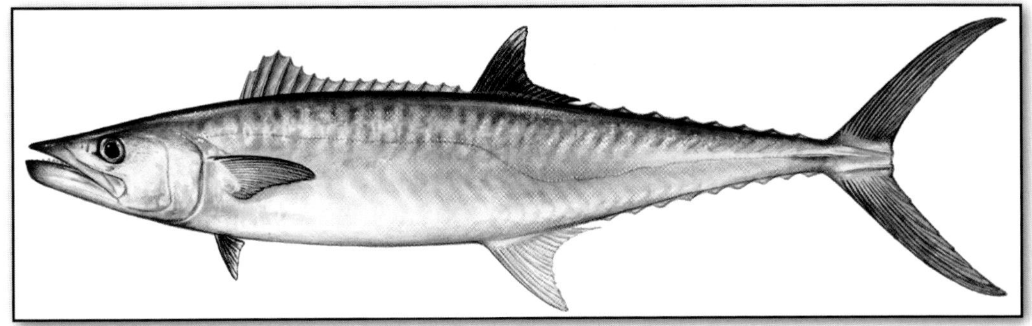

28. King Mackerel *(Scomberomorus cavalla)* page 45

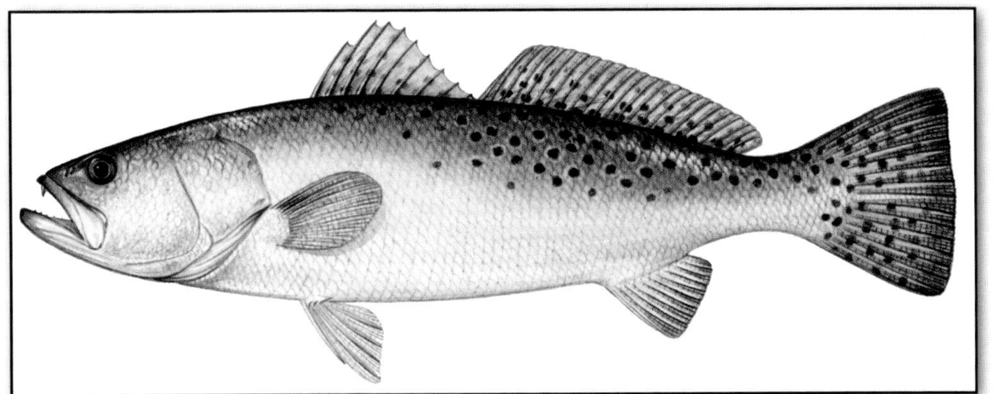

29. Spotted Seatrout *(Cynoscion nebulosus)* pages 8, 57

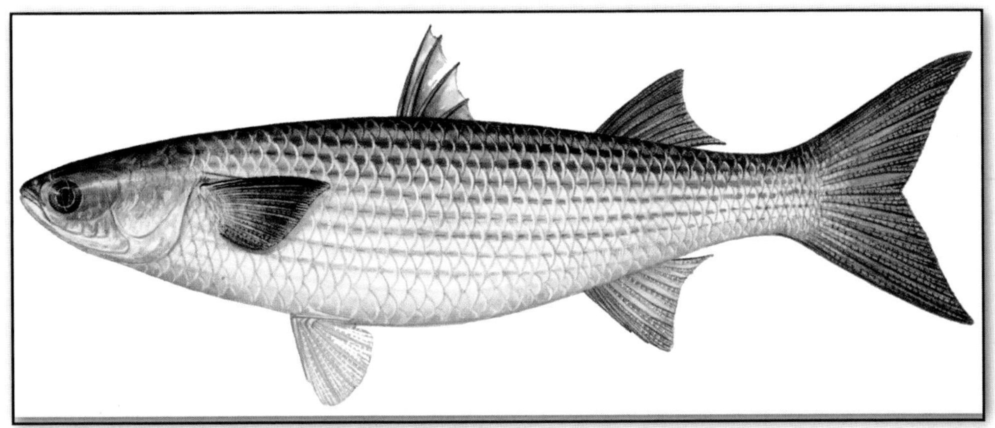

30. Striped Mullet *(Mugil cephalus)* page 57

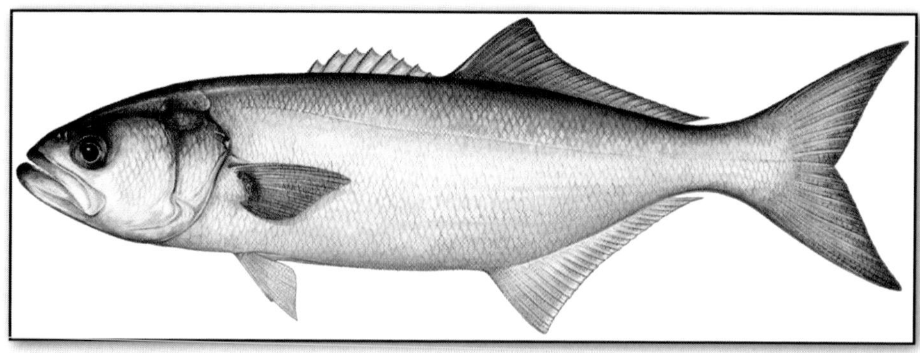

31. Bluefish *(Pomatomus saltatrix)* page 7

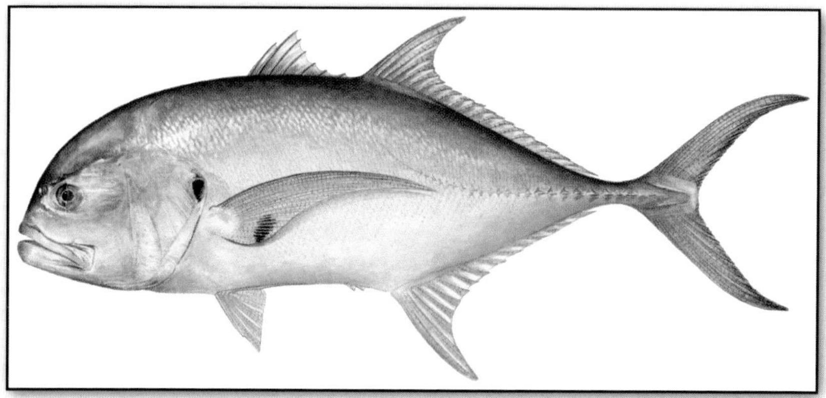

32. Crevalle Jack *(Caranx hippos)* page 40

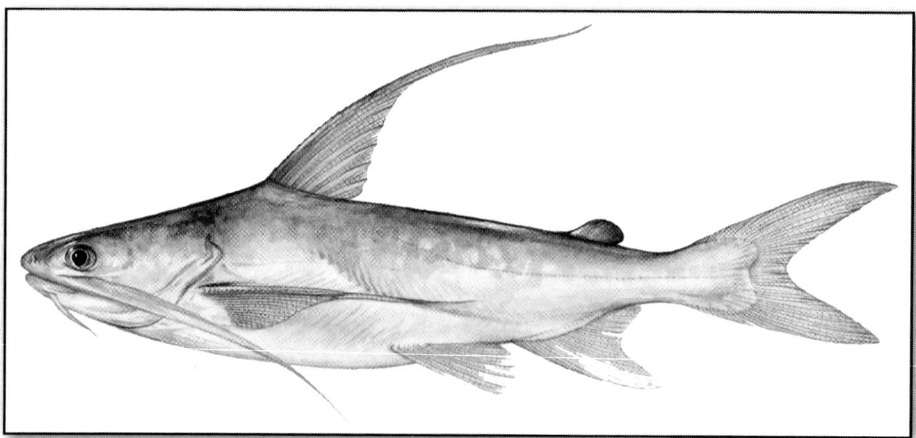

33. Gafftopsail Catfish
(Bagre marinus) page 24

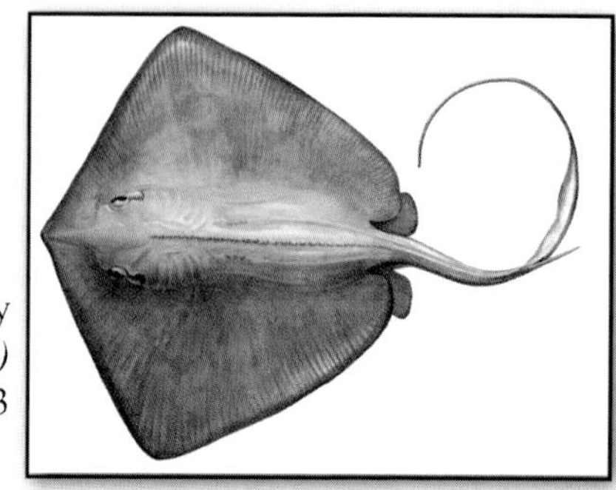

34. Southern Stingray
(Dasyatis americana)
page 23

Ciguatera poisoning

The name "ciguatera" is believed to be derived from the Spanish or Cuban name of "cigua," a commonly eaten Caribbean marine snail *(Cittarium pica)*. Ciguatera has been known since the sixteenth century and has been reported in past years to be poisonous. It is caused by fish and mollusks feeding on toxic algae and accumulating the toxin in their flesh. When these organisms are eaten in quantities by larger fish, the amount of toxin present in their bodies can be considerable. In general, the larger fish are used for human consumption. If they contain the toxin, the consumer may suffer ciguatera symptoms. In this case, get medical attention.

Ciguatera usually occurs in reef or shore fish. It is possible that fish from one area of a reef are poisonous, but not from another nearby area. About three hundred species of fish have been implicated in this type of poisoning (see de Sylva, 1994, and other authors listed at the end of this chapter). Examples discussed in this book are popular commercial and recreational fish, which are generally abundant. Most of them are normally edible. Since there are no outward signs or symptoms to distinguish poisonous from nonpoisonous individuals, this form of fish poisoning is treacherous. In addition, reports of ciguatera intoxications are difficult to authenticate. Seek reliable local knowledge before eating fishes from unfamiliar areas.

Mollusks

Conch, queen conch *(Strombus gigas)*

Range: Bermuda, the Bahamas, southeastern Florida, Caribbean Sea, and southern Gulf of Mexico.

Habitat: Intertidal zone down to 1,200 feet. Sandy areas, grass beds, rubble bottom.

Injury: Presence of ciguatera-like poison in flesh of conch may cause poisoning in humans; symptoms include nausea, vomiting, abdominal pain, weakness, and diarrhea.

Prevention: Avoid eating conch with very heavy or eroded shells. Avoid eating conch from an area where ciguatera is present. Seek local knowledge.

Aid to Victim: No known antidote, treatment is symptomatic. Medical treatment is directed toward eliminating the poison from the body.

Remarks: Reports of poisonous conch are infrequent.

Color plate 4

Fishes

Amberjack, greater amberjack *(Seriola dumerili)*

Range: Tropical and subtropical waters.

Habitat: Open ocean and coastal waters. Occasionally feeding on reefs.

Injury: Ciguatera poisoning, which can be severe. The following symptoms are common: weakness, abdominal pain, vomiting, diarrhea, headache, dizziness, and tingling and numbness of the lips, tongue, and throat. Skin rash, convulsions, and often reversal of feeling of hot and cold may occur.

Prevention: Do not eat large amberjack. The toxin is not destroyed by cooking.

Aid to Victim: No known antidote, treatment is symptomatic. Medical treatment is directed toward eliminating the poison from the body.

Remarks: It is recommended not to eat amberjack in the Leeward Islands of the West Indies. Seek local knowledge before eating amberjack in unfamiliar areas.

Barracuda, great barracuda *(Sphyraena barracuda)*

Range: In the western Atlantic from Massachusetts to southeast Brazil.

Habitat: Inshore wasters and reefs.

Injury: Ciguatera poisoning, which can be severe. The following symptoms are common: weakness, abdominal pain, vomiting, diarrhea, headache, dizziness, and tingling and numbness of the lips, tongue, and throat. Skin rash, convulsions, and often reversal of feeling of hot and cold may occur.

Prevention: Do not eat large barracuda (over 2 pounds). Do not eat fish from areas where ciguatera was recently reported. Seek local knowledge.

Aid to Victim: No known antidote, treatment is symptomatic. Medical treatment is directed toward eliminating the poison from the body.

Remarks: Some recreational fishermen will eat large barracuda despite warnings that they may be toxic. Small barracuda less than 16 inches in total length are generally safe to eat.

Color plate 20

Filefish, fringed filefish *(Monacanthus ciliatus)* **and scrawled filefish** *(Aluterus scriptus)*

Range: From Newfoundland to Florida and the Caribbean, including

Bermuda and northern Gulf of Mexico, south to Argentina.

Habitat: On reefs, usually around benthic plants.

Injury: Ciguatera poisoning, which can be severe. The following symptoms are common: weakness, abdominal pain, vomiting, diarrhea, headache, dizziness, and tingling and numbness of the lips, tongue, and throat. Skin rash, convulsions, and often reversal of feeling of hot and cold may occur.

Prevention: Do not eat fish from areas where ciguatera is reported. Seek local knowledge.

Aid to Victim: No known antidote, treatment is symptomatic. Medical treatment is directed toward eliminating the poison from the body.

Remarks: Other related species may also be affected. Generally, these fish are not desirable as food, although they are eaten in some areas.

Color plate 6

Goatfish, yellow goatfish *(Mulloidichthys martinicus)* **and spotted goatfish** *(Pseudupeneus maculatus)*

Range: Yellow goatfish: In tropical western Atlantic from New Jersey to Rio de Janeiro, including Bermuda, Florida, the Bahamas, and the eastern Gulf of Mexico. Spotted goatfish: New Jersey, Bermuda, and the Bahamas to Brazil. Rare north of Florida.

Habitat: Reefs and grass beds.

Injury: Ciguatera poisoning, which can be severe. The following symptoms are common: weakness, abdominal pain, vomiting, diarrhea, headache, dizziness, and tingling and numbness of the lips, tongue, and throat. Skin rash, convulsions, and often reversal of feeling of hot and cold may occur.

Prevention: Do not eat fish from areas where ciguatera is reported. Seek local knowledge.

Aid to Victim: No known antidote, treatment is symptomatic. Medical treatment is directed toward eliminating the poison from the body.

Remarks: This genus is easily distinguished by two chin barbels.

Color plate 10

Hogfish *(Lachnolaimus maximus)*

Range: Nova Scotia south to Florida, Bermuda, including the Caribbean, and northern Gulf of Mexico to northern South America.

Habitat: Reefs.

Injury: Ciguatera poisoning, which can be severe. The following symptoms are common: weakness, abdominal pain, vomiting, diarrhea, headache, dizziness, and tingling and numbness of the lips, tongue, and throat. Skin rash, convulsions, and often reversal of feeling of hot and cold may occur.

Prevention: Do not eat fish from areas where ciguatera is reported. Seek local knowledge.

Aid to Victim: No known antidote, treatment is symptomatic. Medical treatment is directed toward eliminating the poison from the body.

Remarks: Hogfish are an important food fish in many areas of the Caribbean because of their excellent taste. They are becoming scarce because of spearfishing.

Color plate 13

Jack, crevalle jack *(Caranx hippos)*

Range: Nova Scotia to Uruguay, including the Gulf of Mexico.

Habitat: Inshore waters, around reefs.

Injury: Ciguatera poisoning, which can be severe. The following symptoms are common: weakness, abdominal pain, vomiting, diarrhea, headache, dizziness, and tingling and numbness of the lips, tongue, and throat. Skin rash, convulsions, and often reversal of feeling of hot and cold may occur.

Prevention: Do not eat fish from areas where ciguatera is reported. Seek local knowledge.

Aid to Victim: No known antidote, treatment is symptomatic. Medical treatment is directed toward eliminating the poison from the body.

Remarks: Many jacks have been reported to cause ciguatera poisoning, especially in the northeast Caribbean.

Color plate 32

Moray, green moray *(Gymnothorax funebris)*

Range: New Jersey south to Florida, Bermuda, Caribbean, and northern Gulf of Mexico to Brazil.

Habitat: Reefs, rocky bottom.

Injury: Ciguatera poisoning, which can be severe. The following symptoms are common: weakness, abdominal pain, vomiting, diarrhea, headache, dizziness, and tingling and numbness of the lips, tongue and throat. Skin rash, convulsions, and often reversal of feeling of hot and cold may occur.

Prevention: Do not eat morays, no matter where they are caught.

Aid to Victim: No known antidote, treatment is symptomatic. Medical treatment is directed toward eliminating the poison from the body.

Remarks: Other moray species are implicated in this type of poisoning.

Parrotfish, blue parrotfish *(Scarus coeruleus)*, **midnight parrotfish** *(S. coelestinus)*, **and stoplight parrotfish** *(Sparisoma viride)*

Range: Maryland, Bermuda, and the Bahamas to Brazil. Absent from the northern Gulf of Mexico.

Habitat: Inshore waters and on reefs.

Injury: Ciguatera poisoning, which can be severe. The following symptoms are common: weakness, abdominal pain, vomiting, diarrhea, headache, dizziness, and tingling and numbness of the lips, tongue and throat. Skin rash, convulsions, and often reversal of feeling of hot and cold may occur.

Prevention: Do not eat fish from areas where ciguatera is reported. Seek local knowledge.

Aid to Victim: No known antidote, treatment is symptomatic. Medical treatment is directed toward eliminating the poison from the body.

Remarks: Other parrotfish species are also implicated in causing this type of poisoning.

Color plate 2, 14

Sharks, great white shark *(Carcharodon carcharias)* **and hammerhead shark** *(Sphyrna zygaena)*

Range: From Nova Scotia south in west Atlantic to Argentina.

Habitat: Inshore waters and open ocean.

Injury: Elasmobranch poisoning, thought to be a form of ciguatera poisoning. Nausea, vomiting, abdominal pain, diarrhea, headache, and possibly respiratory distress may occur.

Prevention: Do not eat large sharks from areas where poisoning is reported. Do not eat shark livers.

Aid to Victim: No known antidote, treatment is symptomatic. Medical treatment is directed toward eliminating the poison from the body.

Remarks: The poison is often concentrated in the liver. Although fatalities are known to occur, none have been reported from Florida and vicinity.

Snapper, mangrove or gray snapper *(Lutjanus griseus)* **and schoolmaster** *(L. apodus)*

Range: Massachusetts south to Florida, Bermuda, Caribbean, the Bahamas, and northern Gulf of Mexico to southeast Brazil.

Habitat: These are inshore fish occupying a wide variety of habitats, including mangroves and reefs; sometimes also found in fresh and brackish waters.

Injury: Ciguatera poisoning, which can be severe. The following symptoms are common: weakness, abdominal pain, vomiting, diarrhea, headache, dizziness, and tingling and numbness of the lips, tongue, and throat. Skin rash, convulsions, and often reversal of feeling of hot and cold may occur.

Prevention: Do not eat fish from areas where ciguatera is reported. Seek local knowledge.

Aid to Victim: No known antidote, treatment is symptomatic. Medical treatment is directed toward eliminating the poison from the body.

Remarks: Mangrove snappers generally occur in large schools. The fish may reach 8 to10 pounds.

Color plate 18

Surgeonfish, ocean surgeon *(Acanthurus bahianus)*

Range: Massachusetts to south Florida, including Bermuda, Caribbean, Gulf of Mexico (except northeast) to Brazil. Rare north of Florida.

Habitat: Reefs.

Injury: Ciguatera poisoning, which can be severe. The following symptoms are common: weakness, abdominal pain, vomiting, diarrhea, headache, dizziness, and tingling and numbness of the lips, tongue and throat. Skin rash, convulsions, and often reversal of feeling of hot and cold may occur.

Prevention: Do not eat fish from areas where ciguatera is reported. Seek local knowledge.

Aid to Victim: No known antidote, treatment is symptomatic. Medical treatment is directed toward eliminating the poison from the body.

Remarks: Surgeon fish possess large spines near the tail that can cause injury (see Chapter 6).

Color plate 16

Triggerfish, ocean triggerfish *(Canthidermis sufflamen)*

Range: Massachusetts, Bermuda south to Florida, northern Gulf of Mexico to South America.

Habitat: Open water, reefs.

Injury: Ciguatera poisoning, which can be severe. The following symptoms are common: weakness, abdominal pain, vomiting, diarrhea, headache, dizziness, and tingling and numbness of the lips, tongue, and throat. Skin rash, convulsions, and often reversal of feeling of hot and cold may occur.

Prevention: Do not eat fish from areas where ciguatera is reported. Seek local knowledge.

Aid to Victim: No known antidote, treatment is symptomatic. Medical treatment is directed toward eliminating the poison from the body.

Remarks: The queen triggerfish, *Balistes vetula*, is also suspected of being poisonous in the Caribbean.

Yellowfin grouper *(Mycteroperca venenosa)* **and Nassau grouper** *(Epinephelus striatus)*

Range: Bermuda, Florida, and southern Gulf of Mexico to Brazil.

Habitat: Reefs, also common in deep water.

Injury: Ciguatera poisoning, which can be severe. The following symptoms are common: weakness, abdominal pain, vomiting, diarrhea, headache, dizziness, and tingling and numbness of the lips, tongue, and throat. Skin rash, convulsions, and often reversal of feeling of hot and cold may occur.

Prevention: Do not eat fish from areas where ciguatera is reported. Seek local knowledge.

Aid to Victim: No known antidote, treatment is symptomatic. Medical treatment is directed toward eliminating the poison from the body.

Remarks: The specific name "venenosa" refers to the reputation of that grouper to be more frequently toxic (ciguatera) than are other grouper species.

Color plate 12

Turtles

Hawksbill turtle *(Eretmochelys imbricata)*

Range: Tropical and subtropical ocean waters worldwide. Occasionally found in temperate oceans.

Habitat: Open ocean and nearshore, and on beaches during nesting season.

Injury: Ciguatera-like poisoning. Possibly caused by the turtle's diet consisting of toxic algae. The toxin is retained in the flesh.

Prevention: Seek local knowledge concerning the presence of cases of ciguatera.

Aid to Victim: No known antidote, treatment is symptomatic. Medical treatment is directed toward eliminating the poison from the body.

Remarks: Apparently no authentic cases reported from this area, only in Asia. Note that all sea turtles in U.S. waters and their nests on the beaches are protected and must not be molested or harmed.

Color plate 19

Scombroid poisoning

Scombroid poisoning from mackerels and tunas is different from ciguatera poisoning in that it is caused by bacterial action in the fishes' muscle tissue after death, which produces a poisonous substance called scombrotoxin. According to recent findings, it is not found in fresh fish and therefore can be avoided by icing the catch immediately. The name of this disease came about because originally only tuna and tunalike fishes, including mackerel, bonito, and saury, were linked to the disease. Additional studies demonstrated that at least eight other fish species groups, including such popular species as mahi mahi *(Coryphaena* spp., also known as dolphin fish), bluefish *(Pomatomus saltatrix)*, and salmon *(Oncorhynchus* spp.) are also carriers for this disease. Certain conditions usually are hazardous, including improper shipboard handling of fish, poor storage facilities, and temperatures over 59° F (15° C). The extent of poisoning can be much more severe if the fish also has an off-taste when eaten. Symptoms usually appear a short time after ingestion and may include some or all of these symptoms: cutaneous rash, edema, inflammation of skin, gastrointestinal disturbance (nausea, vomiting, diarrhea), hypotension (low blood pressure), headaches, palpitation, and itching.

Mackerel, king mackerel, kingfish *(Scomberomorus cavalla)*

Range: From Massachusetts to southern Brazil , including northern Gulf of Mexico.

Habitat: Open ocean.

Injury: Scombroid poisoning. The following symptoms are common: redness of the skin, face flushed and swollen, headache, dizziness, circulatory problems, and stomach distress.

Prevention: Fish should be iced as soon as caught. Do not leave your catch in the sun; do not eat fish if it has a "peppery" taste.

Aid to Victim: Antihistamine drugs and other clinical methods.

Remarks: Cases mainly have been reported from the Caribbean. This type of poisoning also has been reported from other members of this family, namely wahoo, Spanish mackerel, and cero mackerel.

Color plate 28

Tuna, skipjack tuna *(Euthynnus pelamis)*

Range: Worldwide. In the western Atlantic, southern Nova Scotia, northern Gulf of Mexico to Brazil.

Habitat: Cosmopolitan in tropical and subtropical waters in the western Atlantic.

Injury: Scombroid poisoning. The following symptoms are common: redness of the skin, face flushed and swollen, headache, dizziness, circulatory problems, and stomach distress.

Prevention: Fish should be iced as soon as caught. Do not leave your catch in the sun; do not eat fish if it has a "peppery" taste.

Aid to Victim: Antihistamine drugs and other clinical methods.

Remarks: Cases have mainly been reported from the Caribbean. Besides affecting skipjack, this poison has been reported from mackerels, wahoo, and possibly other fish (see above).

Tetrodotoxin (puffer poison)

Certain puffer species contain a powerful toxin in the liver, intestines, skin, and reproductive organs. Since it is a very strong poison known to cause fatalities, get medical attention when symptoms occur. For more details on symptoms, see species below. Species causing puffer poisoning are in the family Tetraodontidae (puffers, blowfish, balloon fish). They are small and lack pelvic fins. Their most obvious characteristic is an ability, when disturbed, to inflate themselves to a spheroid form almost twice their size. As mentioned above, the tetrodotoxin is concentrated in certain organs and tissues; ovaries are almost always toxic, and to a somewhat lesser extent, the liver, bile, skin, and flesh. Despite the danger of eating these fish, called fugu, the Japanese are fond of them. Using specially trained cooks who know the proper species to serve and how to butcher them reduces the chance of poisonings. However, Japanese deaths annually attributed to eating puffers vary from a few to the hundreds. Eating fugu is a gamble. In mild doses the toxin reportedly provides a feeling of happiness, warmth, and well-being. As one person reported to his wife shortly before his death, he felt like he "was walking on a cloud." For many years it was believed that puffer fish manufactured their own poison. At this time, a commensal bacterium is thought to be the cause.

Balloonfish *(Diodon holocanthus)* **and porcupinefish** *(D. hystrix)*

Range: The balloonfish is found in Florida and the Bahamas, south to Brazil; northern U.S. limits are uncertain. The porcupinefish is found from Massachusetts to Bermuda, the Gulf of Mexico and south to Brazil.

Habitat: Both species inhabit reefs. The balloonfish is also found in shallow waters.

Injury: Puffer poisoning. Causes lethargy, muscular weakness, dizziness, nausea, numbness, respiratory distress, possibly paralysis in severe cases, and death.

Prevention: Do not eat fish of the family of spiny puffers.

Aid to Victim: There is no known antidote. Treatment is symptomatic. Get medical attention.

Remarks: Both species belong to the family of spiny puffers. In spite of the health hazard, some people still eat puffers. This is dangerous because the intestines, liver, skin, and reproductive organs, which are the sources of the poison, may contaminate the flesh during cleaning. In Asia, this poison is known to cause fatalities from related species.

Color plate 22

Puffer, checkered puffer *(Sphoeroides testudineus)*

Range: Rhode Island, Bermuda south to Florida, and southern Gulf of Mexico to southeast Brazil.

Habitat: Rocky bottom, inshore waters.

Injury: Puffer poisoning. Causes lethargy, muscular weakness, dizziness, nausea, numbness, respiratory distress, possibly paralysis in severe cases, and death.

Prevention: Do not eat puffer fish.

Aid to Victim: No known antidote, treatment is symptomatic. Medical treatment is directed toward eliminating the poison from the body.

Remarks: Despite the health hazard, some people still eat puffers. This is dangerous because the intestines, liver, skin, and reproductive organs, which are the sources of the poison, may contaminate the flesh during cleaning. In Asia, this poison is known to cause fatalities from related species.

Ocean sunfish *(Mola mola)*

Range: All temperate, tropical, and subtropical seas in both the Atlantic and Pacific Oceans. Western Atlantic from Newfoundland to northern South America.

Habitat: From the surface, where the sunfish may be observed lying on its side apparently basking in the sun, down to more than 1,000 feet.

Injury: The species can contain tetrodotoxin and can cause ciguatera poisoning. Cases can be severe. The following symptoms are common: weakness, abdominal pain, vomiting, diarrhea, headache, dizziness, and tingling and numbness of the lips, tongue, and throat. Skin rash, convulsions, and often reversal of feeling of hot and cold may occur.

Prevention: Very few sunfish are captured; most information is obtained from specimens that are sick or dead, floating at the surface. The best rule is never to eat sunfish.

Aid to Victim: No known antidote, treatment is symptomatic. Medical treatment is directed toward eliminating the poison from the body.

Remarks: Sunfish are host to a wide variety of internal and external parasites, with roundworms in the body muscles, giving this flesh a very unappetizing appearance, and providing further reason not to eat the species.

Scrawled cowfish *(Lactophrys quadricornis)* **and trunkfish** *(L. trigonus)*

Range: Massachusetts, Bermuda, and northern Gulf of Mexico to Brazil.

Habitat: Inshore areas, seagrass beds, reefs.

Injury: Pufferlike poisoning, possibly toxic liver. Eating this fish also may cause ciguatera poisoning. Symptoms include weakness, numbness, dizziness, nausea, and respiratory distress.

Prevention: Do not eat any members of the boxfish family, including the cowfish and trunkfish.

Aid to Victim: No known antidote, treatment is symptomatic. Medical treatment is directed toward eliminating the poison from the body.

Remarks: It is curious that anyone would want to eat these fish. Their bodies are encased in a bony covering resembling a trunk (from which the name originated). This armor serves as protection against predators and makes the fish difficult to clean. Some species secrete a toxic substance when disturbed.

Color plate 5

Reproductive products (eggs)

Horseshoe crab *(Limulus polyphemus)*

Range: Maine to Louisiana.

Habitat: Close to shore on sandy bottom and in estuaries.

Injury: There are no reports on the practice of eating the eggs, or roe, of the North American horseshoe crab. However, some relatives of the American horseshoe crab in southeast Asia are considered a delicacy and the viscera, unlaid eggs, or flesh are eaten during the reproductive season. Consuming these eggs can cause poisoning and death. There are a variety of symptoms, including dizziness, headaches, nausea, vomiting, abdominal cramps, diarrhea, cardiac palpitation, numbness of limbs tingling of lower extremities, and decreased body temperature. In severe cases symptoms include the sensation of heat in mouth, throat, and stomach; muscular paralysis; hyper-salivation; drowsiness; and loss of consciousness. Death may occur within approximately sixteen hours after symptoms appear.

Prevention: It is foolhardy to eat any animals or animal products unless there is clear evidence that it is recognized as safe for human consumption.

Aid to Victim: No known antidote, treatment is symptomatic. Medical treatment is directed toward eliminating the poison from the body.

Remarks: The common name "horseshoe crab" is misleading because it is not a crab but a relative of spiders and scorpions.

Sea urchin, long-spined black urchin *(Diadema antillarum)*

Range: Florida and Bermuda to northern South America.

Habitat: Rocky bottom, reefs, grass beds, pilings, and sea walls.

Injury: Sea urchins are a problem for swimmers and waders because of the numerous brittle spines that may puncture the skin and in some cases break off in the flesh. It is questionable whether their gonads (both male and female reproductive organs and their products) are safe to eat. Many sea urchins become toxic because of the toxic algae they feed on. This toxin is believed to concentrate in the gonads. Symptoms are acute gastritis, nausea, vomiting, diarrhea, abdominal pain, and severe headaches.

Prevention: Since many of the marine biotoxins are powerful neurotoxins it is foolhardy to experiment with eating gonads of any sea urchins unless there is reliable information that they are safe to eat.

Aid to Victim: No known antidote, treatment is symptomatic. Medical treatment is directed toward eliminating the poison from the body.

Remarks: Some species of sea urchins are considered an important food in Japan, where they are imported from countries worldwide. Local markets for sea urchins exist in Barbados, West Indies. Gonads of some species are toxic in certain geographic areas and may be toxic at one time but not another; usually they are toxic during the reproductive season. In the Florida Keys, a sudden die-off has led to a drastic reduction in numbers of this species over the past decade. The cause has not yet been determined.

Color plate 21

Species containing pollutants

Because of the effect of human-generated pollution on coastal waters, marine plants and animals may become diseased or die. This is of great ecological concern along the U.S. Atlantic coast. In addition, the possible effect on humans when eating fish and shellfish from polluted areas is of immediate concern, since it is a public health issue.

Untreated or insufficiently treated sewage is one source of pollution. Some shellfish, such as mollusks, take in viruses and bacteria and tend to accumulate the poisons produced by them. These microorganisms and their wastes can cause diseases in humans, including hepatitis (liver inflammation), typhoid fever (bacteria causing cramps and diarrhea), and paralytic shellfish poisoning. Over time, the latter disease has caused deaths in 10 to 25 percent of cases reported. One group of bacteria, *Vibrio*, found in shellfish, causes intestinal disorders in humans. Among the many kinds of wastes that industrial and agricultural areas release into nearby waters and ultimately the sea are pesticides, including persistent chlorinated hydrocarbons, toxic trace metals, detergents, plasticizers, and polychlorinated biphenyls (PCBs). Fish and shellfish can accumulate these pollutants, which in turn will be harmful to the consumer.

The most publicized and serious case of heavy metal poisoning occurred in Japan from 1953 to 1961. There, mercury released from industry was accumulated in the tissues of fish and shellfish. The seafood, used for human consumption, caused the deaths of 46 persons, and 100 or more suffered serious neurological disturbances from chronic poisoning in the year 1953 alone.

Although many other pollutants accumulate in fish and shellfish, at this time the evidence of mercury as a human health hazard is well established, while work on others is ongoing. Needless to say, it is important to avoid eating fish or shellfish from areas known to be contaminated with industrial or domestic pollutants.

Some fish and shellfish may become diseased by pollutants present in the water. These toxic substances may act as irritants on the fish and produce symptoms such as clearly visible skin lesions, protrusions of eyeballs (exophthalmus), fin rot, and possibly tumors and malformations. Fishermen need to realize that diseased animals are unsuitable for consumption. Furthermore, since they have been in contact with toxins, they may have accumulated pollutants in the flesh that would make them poisonous for humans to eat. Do not eat fish from polluted waters, especially near harbors and sewage outfalls. Drainage canals in many coastal states receive domestic, industrial, and agricultural wastes. Fish and shellfish taken from these canals may be contaminated.

Oyster, American oyster *(Crassostrea virginica)*

Range: On the Atlantic Coast of North America from the Canadian Maritimes southward around Florida, and all along the Gulf of Mexico to the West Indies and Venezuela.

Habitat: Mangrove roots, flats, and inshore banks.

Injury: Upset stomach, diarrhea, vomiting, gastrointestinal disturbance, and hepatitis.

Prevention: Do not eat oysters from areas declared unsafe by government authorities.

Aid to Victim: Get medical attention in severe cases.

Remarks: Public health authorities can provide information on safety of local oyster beds. Poor water quality has become a serious problem on Florida's northwest coast, where oyster fisheries had to be closed in the past few years to protect consumers. The source of the problem is bacterial contamination caused by sewage or other man-made pollution in waters surrounding oyster beds.

Reef and estuarine fish (snappers, groupers, grunts, jacks, etc.)

Range: Tropical and temperate waters, Florida, the Bahamas, and northern Gulf of Mexico to Brazil.

Habitat: Inshore on hard bottom, seagrass beds, mangrove creeks, and reefs.

Injury: Possible health disturbances when eating fish containing pollutants.

Prevention: Do not eat fish caught near sources of domestic, industrial or agricultural pollution, including sewage outfalls.

Aid to Victim: Get medical attention.

Remarks: There may be bacterial lesions on the fish such as red spots on fins and body. The amount of pollutants humans can ingest from eating fish without ill effects differs with species and types of pollutants.

Grunts *(Haemulon* spp.)

Range: Bermuda, North Carolina to Florida, the Bahamas, Gulf of Mexico, the Caribbean to Brazil.

Habitat: Grass beds, reefs, and inshore waters.

Injury: Bacterial lesions on the fish. Red spots on fins and body. Bacterial infection caused by sewage pollution may cause serious human illness.

Prevention: Avoid eating fish from known polluted areas.

Aid to Victim: Get medical attention.

Remarks: Do not eat fish from known contaminated waters.

Color plate 15

Species with parasitic diseases

Taste preferences for preparing fish currently range from thoroughly cooked to raw. As part of the menu Japanese restaurants serve raw, lightly cooked, or smoked fish. This is new to Westerners, but a tradition to Asians who have eaten sushi and sashimi for centuries. The change in dietary habits has its downside. In the United States, there are reports of at least fifty cases, most of these since 1980, of parasitic infections from eating improperly prepared marine fish. Although seafood is excellent fare for humans, to avoid possible human health dangers some simple precautions must be taken. Cooking and freezing usually destroys parasites. Microwaving fish for very short periods may not kill potentially harmful parasites.

The parasites of marine fish and shellfish that are important from a human health standpoint include "larger" or macro-parasites such as worms. Often these are roundworms (nematodes) and tapeworms (cestodes), a type of flatworm. Another type of flatworm, the trematode, is also present in marine fish. There is some evidence that those trematodes may infect humans.

The parasites discussed here are normally found encysted in the flesh of fish. Parasites are found in fish in all organs and organ systems, but since most people eat only the flesh, many parasites in other organs are of no concern. However, the roundworms, discussed below, have a nasty habit of leaving the viscera of ungutted herring and mackerel during storage and moving into the flesh.

All of these worms have complicated, indirect life cycles. They parasitize those fish and invertebrates that serve as intermediate hosts between the egg stage and larval stage, until they transform into adult worms and move into a final host where they spend the remainder of their lives. Humans become infected when they eat larval parasites encysted in the flesh of the intermediate that is either uncooked, lightly cooked, or smoked, or has never been frozen.

This section deals only with eating marine fish and with the chance of acquiring parasitic disease. The long history of humans acquiring parasites from freshwater fish in Asia is not discussed here, nor is sickness that may result from improper preservation, from eating fish and shellfish that are naturally toxic from foods they eat, or from natural toxins produced within the bodies of fish.

Fortunately for seafood lovers, most parasites that infect fish and shellfish are harmless to humans, since their bodies do not provide the right conditions for fish parasites to encyst, metamorphose, and reproduce. For a parasite to infect and live in a host, it must be able not only to overcome the physical and chemical defenses of the host, but under specific conditions derive substances from the host for its survival and development. However, unfortunately for humans, several marine parasite species, if given the chance, will infect them with possible pathological consequences. These are usually parasites that have fish as an intermediate host and an adult marine mammal (such as porpoises or seals) as a final host. The importance here is that the environment in the intestinal tract in large aquatic mammals or land mammals is roughly similar to that in humans. This also applies where land mammals such as raccoons or bears may be parasitized by worms from coastal fishes or salmon in rivers and streams. In contrast, the larval tapeworms found in fish such as sea trout have sharks as final hosts, where the conditions are right for transformation into adult parasites. Fortunately, the human intestinal tract is not similar to that of the shark.

In summary, damage done to the health of the host depends on the species of parasite, its size, the numbers present, and the impact on the host's organs. Parasitism is a widespread natural phenomenon. To some extent, we can prevent and control the level of human infection by parasites from domestic animals used for food, but there is little that can be done to prevent wild fish from getting parasites, so protection of public health must come after capture. Cultured marine fish and shellfish may not contain as many parasites as their wild counterparts because the ecosystem on which parasites depend, including the presence of intermediate hosts found in nature, may not be present in aquaculture facilities. The use of artificial foods reduces the chances of parasitic infection of those fishes raised for human consumption.

Since only certain marine fish have parasites potentially harmful to man, this health hazard can be avoided by striking these fish from one's diet. Unfortunately, some very popular fish, such as salmon, herring, and cod, harbor worms. Also, potentially wormy fish may be misidentified, or may completely lose their identity after filleting and passing through market channels. Therefore, it is important to cook fish thoroughly.

Note that most of the species eaten raw in sushi and sashimi are high seas fish, such as tuna, which are known to be safe.

Parasites in fishes

Roundworms (nematodes)

Marine fish are frequently infected with larval roundworms. They are elongate, cylindrical worms tapering at each end, and may be colored white, yellow, brown, or red. Not all worms in this group are harmful to humans, but since knowledge of minor morphological differences between species is required for identification, it is wise to assume that any roundworm found encysted or free in a fish may be a potential human health hazard. They are most commonly found in gadoid fish (cod and haddock) and in herrings, but they infect other fish as well. A case of a live fish nematode in a human was recorded as early as 1876.

As an example of the potential risks from nematodes, people in the Netherlands are fond of eating green herring, which is sold lightly salted. If gutting and salting is delayed until the fishing vessel reaches port, human infections with roundworms can result. It has been found that roundworms can move from the viscera to the musculature during storage on ice, and the light salting that follows is not harmful to the worms. Such movement does not take place in all species infected with this roundworm, but is also known to occur in the mackerel.

Tapeworms (cestodes)

Tapeworms are known to many more people than roundworms. They attach to the host's intestine with a structure called a scolex, and the body consists of a number of similar segments. For some time, fish tapeworms have been recognized as human pathogens in northern Europe. Recently, they have become common in North America. Consumers in western Canada and Alaska become infected by eating raw or undercooked and improperly smoked salmon. The larval worms are encysted in salmon flesh, usually sockeye salmon, which become infected as young fish during their rather long sojourn in fresh water. The first intermediate host is a small freshwater crustacean, which is eaten by the fish as it migrates to the sea; the final host in the ocean is a fish-eating mammal, such as a seal or sea lion. Bears become infected when fishing for salmon spawning in rivers and streams. Bears defecate the tapeworm segments containing eggs, which are then eaten by the crustaceans, which in turn are eaten by young salmon.

There is a chance that these worms may become adults in humans. Symptoms such as abdominal pain, constipation, or diarrhea may characterize infection by the fish tapeworm, but in most cases no symptoms are noted. Unlike the nematodes, the eggs released by the tapeworm in the host's feces permit diagnosis of a tapeworm infection.

Flatworms (trematodes)

The trematodes ("flukes") are also parasites of salmon and may cause human infections when the fish is insufficiently cooked. Cases are recorded in Russia and the west coast of the United States from Washington to northern California. Abdominal pain and diarrhea may be signs of the disease, but occasionally no symptoms occur. However, eggs in the feces of a patient will signal the presence of the parasite.

Leeches

Occasionally leeches, or "blood suckers," seagoing relatives of earthworms, attach to the skin of fishes and are found by fishermen. They are attached so loosely that they may drop off the host when it is caught. Others can easily be removed by the angler when the fish is skinned or scaled. They present no health hazard to humans.

Drum, black drum *(Pogonias cromis)* **and high hat** *(Equetus acuminatus)*

Range: Nova Scotia to northern Mexico, including southern Florida; also southern Brazil to Argentina.

Habitat: Inshore waters, over rocky bottom.

Injury: Tapeworm infection of the fish may lead to human infection. Long ribbonlike white worm larvae occur in the flesh. Some tapeworm larvae can become parasites of man when ingested with raw fish dishes. (This condition has been reported from Japan and Peru.) So far no cases have been reported in humans from this geographic area (see "range" above).

Prevention: Remove the parasites. Cook fish well. Avoid raw fish dishes (ceviche, sashimi, etc.) using this species or others unless prepared by a professional chef.

Aid to Victim: Not applicable.

Remarks: The tapeworms are more often found in fish during the summer.

Color plate 11

Flounder, peacock flounder *(Bothus lunatus)*

Range: Bermuda and Florida and the Bahamas to Brazil.

Habitat: Sandy bottom in coastal waters.

Injury: Accidental infection of humans by roundworms in the fish. The round-bodied worm larvae live in the fish flesh or other organs, either free or encysted. In humans, they can cause enteritis and meningioencephalitis. No cases have been reported from this area (see "range" above).

Prevention: Clean and cook fish well. Avoid eating raw or lightly cooked fish.

Aid to Victim: Get medical attention.

Remarks: More infected fish are reported during the summer. Although humans are not natural hosts for most aquatic fish parasites, it is best to exercise care in the preparation of seafood.

Color plate 8

Grouper, Nassau grouper *(Epinephelus striatus)*

Range: Tropical western Atlantic north to the Carolinas.

Habitat: Rocky bottom, reefs.

Injury: Accidental infection of humans by roundworms in the fish. The round-bodied worm larvae live in the fish flesh or other organs, either free or encysted. In humans, they can cause enteritis and meningioencephalitis. No cases have been reported from this area (see "range" above").

Prevention: Clean and cook fish well. Avoid eating raw or lightly cooked fish. When cleaning the fish remove parasites if in small numbers.

Aid to Victim: Get medical attention.

Remarks: More infected fish are reported during the summer. Although humans are not natural hosts for most aquatic fish parasites, it is best to exercise care in the preparation of seafood.

Color plate 12

Mackerel, Spanish mackerel *(Scromberomorus maculatus)*

Range: Cape Cod to southern Florida, and entire Gulf of Mexico. Absent from the Bahamas and Antilles, except Cuba and Haiti, and rare north of Chesapeake Bay.

Habitat: Open ocean, seasonally in Biscayne Bay, south Florida.

Injury: Tapeworm infection of the fish leading to infection of humans. Long ribbonlike white worm larvae in the flesh of fish ingested with the raw dish "ceviche" have been reported infecting humans in South America and Asia (see symptoms above). Mackerel are often used for this dish. No known infections have been reported from this area (see "range" above).

Prevention: Avoid raw fish dishes (ceviche, sushi, sashimi, etc.) when reports of wormy fish are given. Remove the parasites during cleaning of the fish and cook fish well.

Aid to Victim: Accidental infections require medical attention.

Remarks: More infected fish are reported during the summer. Although man is not a natural host for most aquatic fish parasites, it is best to exercise care in the preparation of seafood.

Mullet, striped mullet, gray mullet *(Mugil cephalus)*

Range: Nova Scotia to Brazil, but absent from the Bahamas and most of the West Indies and Caribbean. Nearly worldwide in warm waters.

Habitat: The species is capable of a wide range of tolerance to temperatures from temperate to tropical waters. Some enter fresh water. Spawning takes place off shore in large schools.

Injury: Infection of the fish with trematodes may lead to human infection. Small cysts are noticeable in flesh, eyes, or other organs of the fish. Trematode infections of man caused by eating raw fish are well known from Asia. Some years ago at least one report from Florida mentioned a trematode from a mullet infecting a child. This was not authenticated. In other areas of the world, injury to humans varies according to the species of trematode infecting the fish.

Prevention: Clean and cook fish well. Avoid eating raw or lightly cooked fish.

Aid to Victim: Get medical attention.

Remarks: More infected fish are reported during the summer. Although humans are not a natural host for most aquatic fish parasites, it is best to exercise care in the preparation of seafood.

Color plate 30

Seatrout, spotted seatrout *(Cynoscion nebulosus)*

Range: Cape Cod southward around the Gulf of Mexico to the Gulf of Campeche, Mexico.

Habitat: Grass beds inshore, in shallow water.

Injury: Tapeworm infection of the fish may lead to infection of humans. Long ribbonlike white worm larvae are imbedded in the flesh. Some tapeworm larvae can become parasites of man when ingested with raw fish. This parasite is reported from Japan and Peru, but no authentic reports are given from North America. This large worm is unappetizing and causes concern to fishermen catching infected fish.

Prevention: Clean and cook fish well. Avoid eating raw or lightly cooked fish.

Aid to Victim: Get medical attention.

Remarks: More infected fish are reported during the summer. Although humans are not natural hosts for most aquatic fish parasites, it is best to exercise care in the preparation of seafood. Clean and cook fish well.

Color plate 29

Snapper, mangrove or gray snapper *(Lutjanus griseus)*

Range: Massachusetts south to the Gulf of Mexico.

Habitat: This is an inshore fish occupying a wide variety of habitats. It is sometimes found in fresh water, and often in brackish water and in marine waters around reefs.

Injury: Infestation of fish by leeches, which are not transferable to humans. Parasitic infestation of the fish with leeches attached to gill area, mouth, and fins may occasionally be seen by anglers. Although unappetizing in appearance, there is no known record of harm to humans.

Prevention: During normal preparation of the fish for cooking, the body parts where the leeches occur will be disposed of. Wash the fish with fresh water.

Remarks: Although humans are not a natural host for most fish parasites, it is best to exercise care in the preparation of seafoods known to harbor parasites.

Snook *(Centropomus undecimalis)*

Range: South Carolina to Texas, south to southern Brazil.

Habitat: Inshore areas, estuaries, bays and inlets.

Injury: Infestation with parasitic crustaceans not transferable to humans. These fish lice (copepods) occur on the body of the fish and give an unappetizing appearance to the fish.

Prevention: Wash the fish with fresh water before filleting or cleaning.

Remarks: Although humans are not natural hosts for most aquatic fish parasites, it is best to exercise care in preparation of seafoods know to harbor parasites.

Color plate 17

Parasites in Crustacea

Although most Americans do not eat raw shrimp, prawns, or crabs, there are records of parasites infecting people who have dined on raw shellfish. Crustaceans serve as hosts for worms similar to those found in fishes and could become potential human health problems. For example, a larval nematode present in warm water shrimp (penaeid shrimp) from the northern Gulf of Mexico can infect laboratory animals such as mice and monkeys. This suggests that humans may be possible hosts, but research results are scarce.

The incidence of infection of humans by crustacean-borne parasites is extremely low in the United States, where cooking is a traditional preparation method. Note that parasites may be killed by freezing (-4°F for 24 hours) or proper cooking (1 minute at 140°F).

Stone crab *(Menippe mercenaria)*

Range: North Carolina, Florida, the Bahamas, through the Gulf of Mexico, including Yucatan and the Greater Antilles.

Habitat: Shallow flats, inshore areas in bays and inlets.

Injury: Trematode infection of the crab, resulting in an unappetizing appearance only, not known to be transferable to humans. This trematode infection is seen as dark spots in the muscles of the host.

Prevention: The parasite is destroyed by cooking. Avoid eating raw or lightly cooked stone crabs.

Aid to Victim: Get medical attention if there is a suspicion of infection.

Remarks: More infected stone crabs are reported during the summer. Although humans are not natural hosts for most aquatic fish and shellfish parasites, it is best to exercise care in the preparation of seafood.

Another stone crab disease that concerns consumers is called shell disease. It results in a discolored, soft, and eroded shell, probably caused by bacteria. Shell disease does not affect the quality of the crabmeat. However, crabs look unappetizing and the disease reduces market value.

Blue crab *(Callinectes sapidus)*

Range: East coast of the U.S. from Massachusetts southward, including Florida and the northern Gulf of Mexico and Texas.

Habitat: Inshore areas in bays and estuaries.

Injury: Pepper spot disease, which appears as small dark spots in the muscles of crabs. It is not known to harm humans. It is caused by an infection of the host by a parasitic protozoan (one-celled animal) leading to an unappetizing appearance.

Prevention: This parasite is destroyed by cooking.

Remarks: Another disease of blue crabs is shell disease, which is caused by bacteria. It is recognizable by discolored, soft, and eroded crab shells. Although there is no threat to human health, it gives crabs an unappetizing appearance and hurts the commercial market. There are no records that either of these diseases adversely affects the quality or flavor of the crabmeat.

Color plate 24

American lobster, northern lobster *(Homarus americanus)*

Range: East coast of North America, from North Carolina to Labrador.

Habitat: From inshore coastal waters over the continental shelf and into deeper waters below the shelf.

Injury: Although not known as harmful to humans, several diseases affect this species. Numerous parasites and diseases occur in northern lobsters, such as species of bacteria (including *Gaffkya homari),* fungi, protozoa, trematodes, nemerteans, acanthocephalans, nematodes, and annelids. Also known are a breakdown of the lobsters' exoskeleton and molt death syndrome (dying during molting). Several diseases cause high mortality to northern lobsters. Examples are red tail (a highly infectious disease causing weakness and death to lobsters, mostly those in confinement); shell disease caused by a bacterium that attacks all parts of the exoskeleton, making the lobster unsightly (it apparently does not enter the flesh and does not affect market value); gas disease, caused by supersaturation of air in aerated water tanks where lobsters are held, resulting in high mortality; and contamination of holding tank waters (fecal wastes of lobsters will kill other lobsters held in confinement). Most lobster diseases do not affect humans, but in an advanced stage will affect marketability and value.

Remarks: Many of the diseases listed above result from catching wild lobsters and holding them in tanks or submerged pens for an extended time.

Additional Reading

Ahmed, F. E. (ed.) 1991. *Seafood Safety.* National Academy Press. Washington, D.C.: 432 pp.

Anderson . D. M. and P. S. Lobel. 1987. The Continuing Enigma of Ciguatera. *Biol. Bull.* 172: 89-107.

Baden, D. G. 1983. Marine Food-Borne Dinoflagellate Toxins. In *International Review of Cytology.* G. H. Bourne and J. F. Danielli (eds.). 82: 99-150. Academic Press, New York.

Baden, D. G. 1989. Brevetoxins: Unique Polyether Dinoflagellate Toxins. *FASEB J.* 3: 1807-1817.

Baden, D. G. 1990. Toxic Fish: Scientists Close in on a Safe Test. *Sea Frontiers.* Internatl. Oceanogr. Foundation. 36(3):8-15.

Baden, D. G., Mende, T. J. , Poli, M. A. and Block, R. E. 1984. Toxins from Florida's Red Tide Dinoflagellate *Ptychodiscus brevis*. In *Seafood Toxins* (E. P. Regelis, ed.). American Chemical Society, Washington, D.C.: 359-367.

de Sylva, D. P. 1963. Systematics and Life History of the Great Barracuda, *Sphyraena barracuda* (Walbaum). Studies in Tropical Oceanography No. 1 Institute of Marine Science, Univ. of Miami Press: 177 pp.

de Sylva, D. P. 1994. Distribution and Ecology of Ciguatera Fish Poisoning in Florida, with Emphasis on the Florida Keys. *Bull. Mar. Sci.* 54(3): 944-954.

de Sylva, D. P. and J. B. Higman. 1979. A Plan to Reduce Ciguatera in the Tropical Western Atlantic Region. *Gulf and Caribbean Fisheries* Institute. 32nd Annual Session: 139-153.

Factor, J. R. (ed.). 1995. *Biology of the Lobster, Homarus americanus.* Academic Press, New York: 528 pp.

Kudo, R. R. 1971. *Protozoology.* Charles C. Thomas, Publisher. Springfield, Illinois: 370-392.

Larson, D. E. (ed.) 1990. *Mayo Clinic Family Health Book.* Food Allergies: 448, 469-471. William Morrow and Co. Inc., New York.

Lutz, R. A. and L. S. Incze. 1979. Impact of Toxic Dinoflagellate Blooms on the North American Shellfish Industry. In *Toxic Dinoflagellate Blooms. Proceeding of the Second International Conference on Toxic Dinoflagellate Blooms, Key Biscayne, Florida.* D. L. Taylor and H. H. Seliger (eds.): 476-483. Elsevier, Amsterdam.

Maran, J. (1991). Legal Implications of Ciguatera (A Case History). In *Ciguatera Seafood Toxins.* D. M. Miller (ed.): 13-20. CRC Press, Boca Raton, FL.

Miller, D. M.(ed.) 1991. *Ciguatera Seafood Toxins.* CRC Press Boca Raton, FL. 176 pp.

Nellis, D. W. and G. W. Barnard. 1986. Ciguatera: A Legal and Social Overview. National Marine Fisheries Service. *Marine Fisheries Review.* 48, (4): 2-5.

Olsen, D. A., D. W. Nellis, and R. S. Wood.1984 Ciguatera in the Eastern Caribbean. *Mar. Fish. Review.* 46 (1): 13-18.

Prudden, T. M. 1962. *About Lobsters.*The Knowlton & McLeary Co. Farmington, Maine: 158 pp.

Risk, Paul H. 1983. *Outdoor Safety and Survival.* John Wiley & Sons, New York: 340 pp.

Rodgers, D. L. and C. Muench. 1986. Ciguatera: Scourge of Seafood Lovers. *Sea Frontiers.* Internal. Oceanogr. Fndn . 32(5): 338-346.

Sindermann, C. J. 1990. *Principal Diseases of Marine Fish and Shellfish. Second Edition. Volume 2. Diseases of Marine Shellfish.* Academic Press, New York: 516 pp.

Sindermann, C. J. 1996. *Ocean Pollution: Effects on Living Resources and Humans.* CRC Press, Boca Raton, Florida: 275 pp.

CHAPTER 4

Pests that Harm Swimmers and Fishermen

Several groups of aquatic organisms causing human health problems do not fit into any of the preceding chapters. Essentially, when these organisms come in contact with swimmers or fishermen they release toxins that irritate skin, form welts and sores, and cause infections. The actual organisms that cause skin irritation may be difficult to determine. Generally, they are common, and include algae, bacteria, protozoa, and larval stages of invertebrates such as jellyfish. The evidence that a certain organism may cause the irritation is often circumstantial; for instance, biologists may confirm the presence of a large population of the suspected organism in the vicinity of an outbreak of aquatic dermatitis.

A few definitions are in order because the organisms in this chapter are very small or microscopic in size. The use of common names on one hand and only scientific names on the other creates confusion. All of the organisms listed below are discussed in this chapter:

Blue-green algae: Marine algae distinguished by the color.

Bacteria: Certain bacteria living on the skin of some fishes can irritate any open sore or wound of a person handling the fish, known as "fish-handler's dermatitis."

Other bacteria, called "flesh-eating" for lack of a better name: They are widely distributed in warm seas and brackish waters. They may cause serious harm to people who come in contact with the bacteria while already in poor health.

Dinoflagellates: These are single-celled organisms that live free in the water. A recently discovered toxic species known only by its scientific name, *Pfiesteria,* kills fish and also produces apparently harmful aerosols.

Fire sponge: This species releases chemical irritants when touched by swimmers.

"Swimmer's itch": This is caused by a free-living larval stage of a parasitic trematode. The larvae may try to penetrate the skin of swimmers in an attempt to find the true final host.

Algae

Blue-green alga *(Lyngbya majuscula)*

Range: Hawaiian Islands (windward side of the islands). The alga also occurs in the Caribbean Sea. Whether it is a cause of dermatitis in the Caribbean has not yet been established.

Habitat: Widespread in open waters.

Injury: The alga contains irritants that produce erythema, blisters, a burning sensation, and necrosis, usually during the summer. Irritation may last for several days. Swimmers come in contact with the floating algae that release the irritants.

Prevention: Follow the advice of lifeguards regarding presence of dermatitis-causing organisms in swimming areas.

Aid to Victim: Get out of the salt water and take a freshwater shower as soon as possible.

Remarks: It has been speculated that ingestion of edible seaweeds contaminated with these algae could increase the chances of gastrointestinal cancer. However, no evidence has been reported that the irritants in *L. majuscula* are responsible for cancer in humans. A species of *Lyngbya* in the Florida Keys is not known to irritate swimmers, snorkelers, and divers.

Bacteria

Erysepeloid bacterium ("fish handler's dermatitis") *(Erysepelothrix insidiosa)*

(Common names include fish shingles, felons, erysepeloid, and fish rose)

Range: The bacterium is widely distributed in the open sea.

Habitat: On crabs, crayfish, and the skin of some fishes, especially scombroid species (tuna, etc.).

Injury: Bacteria living on the skin and mucus of some fishes and invertebrates can irritate any open sore or wound a person may have. Simply handling the catch can cause this irritation in some individuals. Fishermen and workers in fish processing plants are more subject to this type of infection due to exposure while handling fish. A version of this disease originates on the hands or fingers as a sharply defined red area around the site of infection, and is limited to that area. This is usually accompanied by itching, prickling, and pain. An aching or burning sensation may be severe enough to interfere with the patient's sleep. Other symptoms may show a lesion that will become purulent (containing or discharging pus). Yet other types may only cause an annoyance and mild discomfort for a short time.

Prevention: Handling fish with rubber gloves, especially if there is an open wound or cut. Use great care in cleaning species with spines.

Aid to Victim: Treat with corticosteroid cream. Erythromycin ointment should also be applied in cases where the skin is infected, denuded, or has fissures.

Remarks: Apparently the fish on which the bacteria live suffer no harmful effects. This disease has been known for as long as people have been catching and eating fish. It can be an occupational hazard and cause commercial fishermen and fish processors to lose several weeks of work. (See *Atlas of Aquatic Dermatology*, A. A. Fisher, 1978.)

"Flesh-eating" bacterium *(Vibrio vulnificus)*

Range: In warm coastal areas. Most abundant when the temperature is above 70° F.

Habitat: In the water column in full strength seawater or brackish water.

Injury: Human infections will develop if the skin is punctured by sea shells or spines from invertebrates such as sea urchins or blue crabs. Within a short time, perhaps twelve to twenty-four hours after contact with these bacteria, symptoms of chills, leg pain, vomiting, and diarrhea persist as the bacterial infection spreads through the person's body. People with the greatest risk of infection are those who have a weakened immune system or serious illness.

Prevention: Individuals at risk should refrain from wading unprotected or swimming in seawater and from eating raw oysters (see also Chapter 3).

Aid to Victim: The vibrio bacteria can be controlled by antibiotics if treatment is administered very soon after infection.

Remarks: More vibrio-related infections are reported from Florida waters than other coastal areas. Healthy individuals, even if they spend considerable time in the sea, need not worry about infection from this bacterium.

Dinoflagellate *(Pfiesteria piscicida*, also spelled *Pfiesteria piscidia)*

Range: Extending from Delaware Bay south along the east coast of the United States to St. Johns River Estuary. In addition, a second dinoflagellate, not identified to species, has been reported from South Carolina, Florida (St. Johns Estuary, the Indian River, and Pensacola), and Mobile, Alabama.

Habitat: Estuaries.

Injury: Fishermen and divers have reported open sores on their bodies and complained of feeling faint, some experiencing memory loss when they were handling dead fish or were in waters fouled by dead fish. Scientists culturing this dinoflagellate in laboratories reported severe neurological symptoms when they inhaled toxins from cultures. However, the symptoms described are still being debated by some medical personnel who have treated fishermen and divers exposed to aerosols from a fish kill. The toxin released by *P. piscicida* has been linked to large-scale fish kills in an area around Pamlico Sound, North Carolina, and the Pamlico River and Neuse River Estuaries.

Prevention: It is advisable to leave an estuarine area where there is evidence of a fish kill. If a person is downwind of a fish kill, aerosols produced by *P. piscicida* could be harmful. It is also advisable not to handle dead or moribund fish in an area of a fish kill, and lastly, not to eat fish from such an area, no matter how healthy they may appear. While effects on humans from these dinoflagellates vary from person to person, these suggestions appear to be the most prudent way to avoid becoming a victim.

Aid to Victim: At this writing, physicians have been unsure which type of treatment to prescribe. Regarding the scientists who were victims of the symptoms described above, a long rest period seemed to be the way to return to normal.

Remarks: Worldwide, over forty marine dinoflagellates have been found to produce toxins that may cause fish kills. One of the best known is "red tide." The organism actively attacks fish by production of an exotoxin. It narcotizes the fish, which sloughs off the epidermis, and causes open ulcerative lesions. *P. piscicida* then consumes bits of epidermal tissue and blood cells from the dead or dying fish.

Dinoflagellate (*Cryptoperidiniopsis*, a new genus)

Range: Maryland, North Carolina, Florida

Habitat: Warm or temperate brackish waters.

Injury: Fishermen and divers have reported open sores on their bodies and have complained of feeling faint, some of experiencing memory loss when they were handling dead fish or were in waters fouled by dead fish. Scientists working in laboratories culturing this dinoflagellate have reported severe neurological symptoms when they inhaled toxins from cultures. However, the symptoms described have been questioned by some medical personnel who have treated fishermen and divers exposed to aerosols from a fish kill.

There is a single report of a castnet fisherman who put the net leads in his mouth prior to casting (this is a standard technique when deploying the cast net). His catch consisted of mullet with numerous sores on their bodies. Soon afterward lesions developed on his lips and tongue. The similarity of this species to *Pfiesteria* (see above), which is known to harm humans, suggests *Cryptoperidiniopsis* may be a toxic species.

Prevention: As a general rule, avoid any fish with lesions or areas where fish kills have occurred. After handling any sick fish with lesions or large sores, authorities recommend sanitizing hands with a dilute bleach solution.

Aid to Victim: Physicians have been unsure which type of treatment to prescribe. Regarding the scientists who were victims of the symptoms described above, a long rest period seemed to be the way to return to normal.

Remarks: The exact classification of this species and its biology and ecology are unknown. These dinoflagellates with complex life histories are very difficult to identify, and therefore difficult to study and determine their possible toxicity to humans.

Parasites

"Swimmer's itch" *(Austrobilharzia variglandis)* **parasitic flatworm larvae**

Range: Worldwide

Habitat: Beaches, shallow water. Occurs mostly in fresh water, but occasionally also in brackish waters.

Injury: A skin rash or dermatitis. Causative agent is a free-living larval stage of a trematode parasite that can irritate a swimmer's skin by trying to penetrate it. The parasite is actively searching for its normal final host, an aquatic bird, and swimmers are accidentally attacked.

Prevention: Do not swim in areas lifeguards or others list as having an outbreak of swimmer's itch. Leave the water at first sign of skin irritation.

Aid to Victim: Apply alcohol.

Remarks: Wong et al. (Seabather's Eruption. Clinical, histologic, and immunologic features. 1994) point out that "swimmer's itch" differs from seabather's eruption in that it has worldwide distribution, occurs primarily in fresh water, is limited to exposed areas of the body, and caused by schistosomal cercariae, larvae of bird parasites.

Additional Reading

Baden, D. G. 1990. Toxic Fish: Why They Make Us Sick. *Sea Frontiers.* International Oceanographic Foundation: 36 (3): 8-15.

Barker, R. 1997. *And the Waters Turned to Blood.* Simon & Schuster, New York: 346 pp.

Drayton, G. E. 1983. Aquatic Skin Disorders, 260-269. *Management of Wilderness and Environmental Emergencies.* In Auderbach, P. S. and Geehr, E. C. (eds.). Macmillan Publishing Co., New York.

Dunn, D. F. 1982. Menacing Medusae, Horrible Hydroids, and Noxious Cnidarians. *Oceans* (2): 16-23.

Falconer, I. R.(ed). 1993. *Algal Toxins in Seafood and Drinking Water.* Academic Press, Inc., San Diego, CA: 224 pp.

Farlow, J. S., and C. King. 1994. Experts Put Warning on More Than Oysters. *Fathom.* 6(1): 15-16.

Fisher, A. A. 1978. *Atlas of Aquatic Dermatology.* Grune and Straton Publishers, New York: 113 pp.

Moore, R. E. 1984. Public Health and Toxins from Marine Blue-Green Algae. In *Seafood Toxins* E. P. Ragelis, (ed.): 369-376. American Chemical Society, Washington, D.C.

Noga, E. J., S. A. Smith, J. M. Burkholder, C. W. Hobbs, and R. A. Bullis. 1993. A New Ichthyotoxic Dinoflagellate: Cause of Acute Mortality in Aquarium Fishes. *Vet. Rec.* 133: 96-97.

Noga, E. J., L. Khoo, J. B. Stevens, Z. Fan, and J. M. Burkholder. 1996. Novel Toxic Dinoflagellate Causes Epitdemic Disease in Estaurine Fish. *Marine Pollution Bulletin:* 32: 219-224.

Osment, L. S. 1976. Update: Sea Bather's Eruption and Swimmers's Itch. *Cutis* 18: 545-547.

Reichenbach-Klinke, H.H. 1973. Fish Pathology: *A Guide to the Recognition and Treatment of Diseases and Injuries of Fishes, with Emphasis on Environment and Pollution Problems.* T. F. H. Publications Inc, Ltd., Hong Kong: 512 pp.

Sindermann, C, J. 1990. *Principal Diseases of Marine Fish and Shellfish. Vol. 1 Diseases of Marine Fish.* Academic Press, New York: 521 pp.

Torpey, J.and R. M Ingle. 1966. The Red Tide. *State of Florida Board of Conservation.* Educ. Series No. 1: 27 pp.

Wong, D. E., T. L. Meinking, L. B. Rosen, D. Taplin, D. J. Hogan, and J. W. Burnet. 1994. Seabather's Eruption. Clinical, histologic, and immunologic features. *J. American Academy of Dermotology.* 30 (3): 399-406.

CHAPTER 5

Toxic Mucus-Secreting Species

Some fish and other types of marine organisms secrete mucus or foam from glands in their skin. The function of mucus is threefold. It serves as protection for the epidermis, it blocks live bacteria from entering the epidermal cells, and it may reduce friction of swimming through the water. The latter advantage is perhaps of minor benefit to the fish except under certain circumstances, such as rapid bursts of speed to capture a prey organism or to avoid capture. In a few species, mucus is used for cocoon building, nest building, or forming an envelope around themselves when they rest at night. The slimy coating of fishes comes from epidermal cells that are unicellular mucus glands. Large amounts of water can be absorbed by mucus, which is composed almost entirely of glycoproteins (simple proteins bound to carbohydrates).

This slime or foam is toxic if ingested. For this reason, the species discussed in this chapter are best not eaten. In any case, it is imperative that they be carefully skinned and the internal organs removed since they may be highly toxic. The liver, brain, gonads (reproductive organs), and visceral organs are occasionally toxic in some species that are otherwise edible. If the mucus or foam of these organisms comes in contact with the eyes or other sensitive skin areas of the person touching or handling them, irritation may result. In this case, rinse thoroughly and get medical attention.

Sponges

Sponge, fire or red sponge *(Tedania ignis)*

Range: West Indies, Florida.

Habitat: Grass flats or hard bottom, mangrove roots.

Injury: Touching fire sponges may cause a stinging sensation, itching, pain, welts, swelling, or skin reaction similar to poison ivy. Chemical irritants are released by the sponge upon contact. The spicules apparently do not pierce the skin.

Prevention: Beware of all red- or orange-colored sponges. Avoid contact and wear gloves when diving or snorkeling.

Aid to Victim: Soak in dilute acetic acid (commercial white vinegar) or use antiseptic dressings.

Remarks: Fire sponges are easily recognized by their bright red or orange color.

Fishes

Cowfish, scrawled cowfish *(Lactophrys quadricornis),* **and honeycomb cowfish** *(L. polygonia)*

Range: Scrawled cowfish: from Massachusetts and Bermuda to Brazil. Honeycomb cowfish: from New Jersey to Brazil, excluding the Gulf of Mexico.

Habitat: Inshore areas, reefs, and seagrass beds.

Injury: Toxic mucus or foam from the skin of these species may come in contact with the eyes or other sensitive skin of the handler, and may cause irritation.

Prevention: Avoid all contact with cowfish.

Aid to Victim: Rinse affected area thoroughly with fresh water and get medical attention.

Remarks: Anglers and net fishermen should handle these fish with care and wear plastic or rubber gloves.

Color plate 5

Atlantic hagfish *(Myxine glutinosa)*

Range: Coasts of the North Atlantic, from Canada to North Carolina.

Habitat: Generally offshore on muddy or sandy bottom, about 100 to 3,000 feet deep, with temperatures as low as 50° F (10° C).

Injury: The mucus of hagfish has been reported as toxic. Bacterial contamination may be the cause of these reports. In any case, the effect is rather mild irritation of the skin. Hagfish possess numerous glands along both sides of the body, which emit copious quantities of tenacious slime, perhaps for self-defense. (Comments on the amount of mucus produced may be exaggerated and out of proportion to the size of the fish.)

Prevention: Avoid all contact with hagfish. Use gloves to remove hagfish from fishing gear.

Aid to Victim: If irritation is experienced, rinse thoroughly with fresh water. If it should persist, get medical attention.

Remarks: This species presents a serious problem to fishermen because of the damage it does to their catch. The commercial food fish hooked or gilled may have their body cavities completely eaten out by hagfish. As one author put it, this leaves the fishermen with only a bag of bones.

A related species, the Gulf hagfish, occurs in the northeastern Gulf of Mexico at a depth of about 1,500 feet.

Greater soapfish *(Rhypticus saponaceus)*

Range: In the western Atlantic, Bermuda, Florida, the Bahamas, southward to Brazil.

Habitat: Found in shallow water (less than 150 feet) generally over limestone, mixed sand and rocks, and around reefs.

Injury: From its skin, this species releases large amounts of mucus containing a toxic protein. When disturbed or handled by fishermen the mucus turns into a soapy foam, which can cause skin irritation.

Prevention: This slime or foam is also toxic if ingested. If any of the species of fishes described in this chapter are to be eaten, it is imperative that they are methodically skinned and the internal organs removed since those may be toxic.

Aid to Victim: If in the course of handling these fishes, mucus or foam comes in contact with the eyes or other sensitive skin areas of the person cleaning the fish, rinse thoroughly, wash with fresh water, and get medical attention.

Remarks: Due to their small size (usually less than 12 inches), soapfish may be subject to heavy predation. The toxic mucus is thought to be a defense against soapfish predators.

Ocean sunfish *(Mola mola)*

Range: All temperate, tropical, and subtropical seas in both the Atlantic and Pacific Oceans. In the Western Atlantic from Newfoundland to northern South America.

Habitat: From a depth of 1,500 feet to the surface water of open ocean, where the sunfish may be observed lying on its side, apparently basking in the sun.

Injury: Although the ocean sunfish is covered with a thick layer of tough mucus, there are no known reports of harm due to handling these large fish (they may reach over 10 feet in length and weigh more than 5,000 pounds).

Prevention: Since few sunfish are captured, most information is obtained from specimens that are sick or dead, and floating at the surface. The best rule is never to eat sunfish.

Remarks: Aside from the mucus the fish secretes, sunfish are host to a wide variety of internal and external parasites, with roundworms in the body muscles giving this flesh a very unappetizing appearance and further reason not to eat the species.

Amphibia

Marine toad *(Bufo marinus)*

Range: Amazon Basin north to coastal Texas, including Florida.

Habitat: The species lives in supratidal areas in underground burrows during the dry season. It comes out to feed and breed during wet weather (in Florida, May and June).

Injury: Large glands on the body behind the eyes release a milky substance called bufotenine when the toad is frightened or attacked. The toxin is capable of killing a dog, and may cause serious illness to a small child. If the substance comes in contact with a person's eyes, severe irritation will result.

Prevention: Do not handle marine toads and keep pets and children away from them.

Aid to Victim: If a pet cat or dog is biting or mouthing a marine toad, remove the toad with heavy gloves or a heavy towel. Rinse the pet's mouth with a garden hose, without choking the animal. Veterinarians may choose to inject the pet with an antidote and drugs to reduce swelling and calm it down. If children touch toads, wash their hands thoroughly and consult a dermatologist.

Remarks: The species was introduced into Florida to battle insects in the 1930s and 1940s. During 1955, an animal importer released a shipment of one hundred marine toads in Miami-Dade County, Florida. Marine toads may reach the size of a "dinner plate" (5 to 9 inches in length) and weigh about 1 pound. Despite the dangerous consequences of handling marine toads, there are reports that bufotenine is used for its hallucinogenic properties.

Additional Reading, Chapter 5

Edstrom, A. 1992. *Venomous and Poisonous Animals.* Krieger Publishing Company, Malabar, Florida: 210 pp.

Fischer, W. (ed). 1978. FAO Species Identification Sheets for Fishery Purposes: *Western Central Atlantic (Fishing Area 31). Food and Agriculture Organization of the United Nations, Rome.* Vol II.

Fisher, A. A. 1978. *Atlas of Aquatic Dermatology.* Grune and Straton Publishers, New York: 113 pp.

Jensen, D. 1966. The Hagfish. *Sci. Am.* 214 (2): 82-90.

Jorgensen, J.M. et al. (eds.) 1998. *The Biology of Hagfishes.* Chapman & Hall, New York.

Lutz, B. 1971. Venomous Toads and Frogs. Chapter 37. In: Bücherl, W. and E. E. Buckley. *Venomous Animals and their Venoms.* Academic Press, New York. 2: 423-473.

CHAPTER 6

Flying Fish, Fish Beak Injuries, and Fish Processing Injuries

Flying fish *(Cypselurus* spp.)

Range: New England, Florida and the north coast of the Gulf of Mexico south to Brazil.

Habitat: Mostly open ocean, but they move close to islands to spawn. Young may be found in bays. Generally, they are found in tropical and subtropical waters.

Injury: Flying fish commonly reach a length of 1 to 1.5 feet. Because of the oddity of fish that fly, their behavior has received considerable scientific attention. The flights are very short, lasting only seconds, and usually are just above the water's surface. However, some estimates show that under certain conditions of wind and waves, they may rise 20 to 30 feet above the water and land on vessels' decks. There are reports of sailors struck by flying fish, but usually little harm results. Most of these reports are old and occurred on rather slow-moving ships. Today's boaters with high-speed open boats being struck by large flying fish could conceivably lose control of the boat, but the probability of this happening is rather remote.

Prevention: About the only way to avoid the remote possibility of being struck by flying fish is to slow down when individual fish are seen flying in the front of an approaching vessel. It is especially hard to spot them at night when they may be at the surface searching for food.

Aid to Victim: In nearly all reports of flying fish colliding with sailors, the harm to the humans is very limited and usually requires little or no first aid.

Remarks: The flights of flying fish are possible because those species with large rigid pectoral and caudal fins have the ability to skip along the surface and actually glide for extended distances.

Houndfish *(Tylosurus crocodilus)*

Range: New Jersey to Brazil. Found in tropical and warm-temperate waters worldwide.

Habitat: Occurs near or at the surface in coastal waters. The houndfish is a member of the needlefish family, a surface feeder.

Injury: Under certain conditions, houndfish have a habit of jumping over objects floating on the surface of the water. Surf boarders and windsurfers have been injured by this activity, since the fish may reach 5 feet in length and weigh 10 pounds. According to Robins (1986), the large size of the species, the sharp closed jaws that form a swordlike beak, and the leaping habit make this a dangerous fish, especially for persons in small boats using lights at night. Serious wounds and some fatalities have occurred when leaping houndfish have accidentally impaled fishermen. Randall (1960) labeled the houndfish "The Living Javelin" and recounts examples of boaters being struck by the beaks of houndfish, including two accounts of boaters hit in the neck and others hit in the face and in the leg. Deaths have also been recorded. Most confirmed accounts of houndfish accidents are from the Caribbean where many night fisheries are carried out using small skiffs and lanterns. Interviews from small-scale fishermen say that injuries from houndfish are infrequent.

Prevention: Houndfish seem to be startled by lights at night. A bright light shone above the surface of the water may encourage fish in the area to jump and splash near the surface. It is wise to leave the area if this behavior is observed. Houndfish are generally more abundant in shallow water near shore. A sturdy wooden or metal shield placed between the fishermen and the light provides protection from the fish. If a fish lands in the boat it is best thrown overboard as soon as possible.

Aid to Victim: Nearly all cases require medical treatment as soon as possible. Stemming the flow of blood from the wound is an important first aid measure.

Remarks: More water use for recreation purposes such as windsurfing and surfboarding may increase the injuries inflicted by houndfish. Accounts of houndfish in windsurfing areas in Biscayne Bay, Florida, have become more frequent recently. Accidents have not been widely publicized.

Billfish *(Tetrapturus* spp.), **sailfish** *(Istiophorus platypterus),* **and blue marlin** *(Makaira nigricans)*

Range: Worldwide in tropical and warm waters.

Habitat: Billfish generally stay offshore, away from land, except where deep dropoffs occur close to the coast.

Injury: Anyone who has witnessed the fight of large billfish when hooked knows that the long spear is shaken violently from side to side, providing ample warning to fishermen to keep their distance. (The blue marlin can weigh well over 1,500 pounds.) There are numerous accounts of accidents involving humans and billfish.

Prevention: Be extremely careful when attempting to bring a large hooked billfish aboard a vessel.

Aid to Victim: Usually, the wounds incurred by fishermen require medical attention.

Remarks: The speed (as high as 40 to 50 mph) and power of these fish are demonstrated by embedded spears found in the hulls of vessels with both wooden and copper-clad hulls. The most logical explanation for these "attacks" on boats is that the billfish are feeding on small prey fish underneath slow moving boats, logs, or other large floating objects and because of their high speed, large size, and difficulty in maneuvering, they accidentally strike the boat hull. Billfish frequently have been observed to swim rapidly into a school of prey fish while moving their head and body describing a small arc. This behavior has been interpreted as a method of "slashing" the fish in the school and then returning to feed on the dead and injured.

Swordfish *(Xiphias gladius)*

Range: In the western Atlantic from Nova Scotia southward to Argentina.

Habitat: Surface waters to great depths (650 to 2,000 feet) in tropical and temperate waters offshore and near coasts.

Injury: Swordfish reach weights over 1,000 pounds and are equipped with a large sword that can do considerable harm to fishermen. Recent evidence shows that the swordfish uses the sword for laterally slashing schools of fish to obtain food. Unlike bills on billfishes (marlin and sailfish), swords on swordfish are dorsoventrally flattened like a paddle, making this method of food capture efficient. Like the billfishes, there are records of "attacks" on vessel hulls and even a record of one on a submersible. Sport fishermen who fish only occasionally are especially susceptible to physical harm, more than are commercial fishermen who have considerable experience and proper equipment to handle these large fish.

Prevention: Be extremely careful when attempting to bring large hooked swordfish aboard a vessel.

Aid to Victim: Usually the wounds incurred by fishermen are severe and require medical attention.

Remarks: This large, powerful fish may reach a length of 14 feet or more.

Surgeonfish, ocean surgeon *(Acanthurus bahianus)*

Range: Massachusetts, Bermuda, Florida, Gulf of Mexico to Brazil.

Habitat: Reefs of the Western Atlantic.

Injury: Surgeonfish have two spines, one on each side of their caudal peduncle (just forward of the tail fin). When the fish is frightened, the spines are erected and the tail is moved quickly toward an enemy. Anyone who handles these fish carelessly risks severe cuts.

Prevention: Avoid any contact with surgeonfish while diving. If one is hooked on a fishing line, cut the fishing leader rather than trying to unhook the fish.

Aid to Victim: Usually, the wounds incurred by anyone handling surgeonfish are severe and require medical attention.

Remarks: Surgeonfish are frequently displayed in public marine aquaria; aquarium personnel should exercise caution in feeding or handling these fish.

Color plate 16

Collecting shark jaws

Dried shark jaws are sought after as souvenirs of fishing trips and to display as trophies. Also, marine biologists studying shark biology require positive identification of the species they study, which includes the numbers and shapes of teeth. Since many of the sharks and rays are too large to preserve or transport to one's laboratory, they remove the jaws. In the process of removing and cleaning the jaws, severe cuts to hands can result since the teeth are numerous and razor-sharp. Even heavy gloves may be inadequate to avoid painful wounds. If not treated promptly, bacterial infections can develop. Infections are usually more severe and difficult to heal with antibiotics if the shark has been dead for some time.

Handling and processing shark skin

The scales of sharks have characteristic sharp denticles which make handling of the fish and processing of shark skins hazardous. Shark fisheries have increased lately, as well as recreational fishing because of the sharks' strength and ferocity. Heavier fishing pressure increases the chances of a greater number of injuries sustained by humans, unless proper care is taken.

In some areas, fishermen are encouraged to fish for sharks due to overfishing of traditional recreational fish species. Commercial fishermen catch sharks for food, utilizing the flesh (mako, nurse sharks), fins for making shark fin soup, hides for making good quality non-cracking leather, and teeth for jewelry. Marketing shark cartilage for possible cancer control in humans has become popular. Some ten years ago, researchers at the Massachusetts Institute of Technology in Cambridge found a substance that strongly inhibits growth of new blood capillaries that feed tumors, rather than acting directly on tumor growth itself.

Because of the sudden interest in sharks in recent years, they have been threatened by overfishing in some parts of the world. As a result their numbers have declined rapidly, disrupting the natural balance of predator-prey relationships in these areas.

Additional Reading

Beaumariage, D. S. 1968. Commercial Shark Fishing and Processing in Florida. *Florida Board of Conservation.* Ed. Series No. 16: 21 pp.

Fischer, W. (ed.) 1978. FAO Species Identification Sheets for Fishery Purposes, Western Central Atlantic. Fishing Area 31, Sharks, Vol. V. *Food and Agriculture Organization of the United Nations, Rome.*

Hardy, A. 1959. *The Open Sea. Part II: Fish and Fisheries.* Collins, St James Place, London: 322 pp.

Randall, J. E. 1960. The Living Javelin. *Sea Frontiers* . International Oceanographic Foundation. 6(4): 228-233.

Randall, J. E. 1968. *Caribbean Reef Fishes.* TFH Publications, Inc. Neptune, N. J.: 318 pp.

Robins, C. R. et al. 1986. *A Field Guide to Atlantic Coast Fishes of North America.* Houghton Mifflin Co. New York: 354 pp.

CHAPTER 7

Human/Animal Interactions

This chapter addresses the recent trend of humans interacting with animals in the wild or contained in pens or large tanks. Feeding them and/or swimming with them are popular, as are petting aquaria for children.

A number of marine aquaria, and occasionally marine tour operators, entertain visitors by inviting them to interact directly with large aquatic species such as porpoises and certain fishes. This can be a risky business for the untrained. The practice is controversial. In the case of aquaria, proponents say they are educating people, giving them an opportunity to see certain animals "up close." Opponents object for ethical reasons. They especially object to feeding fish in the wild, since it teaches fish to become habituated to handouts rather than to obtain food on their own, as they would in nature. In addition to developing dependence on being fed, aggressive behavior by the animals, which may be hungry, can occur if they are not fed when expected. In the marine environment, if divers feed fish on coral reefs, as some do, reef ecology is disrupted. News stories of large marine animals interacting dangerously with humans invading their territory, describing human injuries and deaths, cannot go unnoticed. The simple fact is that, under these circumstances, the behavior of a wild animal is unpredictable.

Morays deserve special mention because of contradicting reports concerning their behavior. Long thought to be aggressive, they more recently have been described as "gentle." Experienced divers and professional underwater photographers believe that neither description fits the morays. They almost never make unprovoked attacks on divers, but careless human behavior may provoke them. Especially the larger species should be regarded with caution, as one would any wild animal with certain natural instincts and behavior patterns. When humans invade their habitat, marine organisms may react unpredictably.

Interacting with animals in aquaria

Several unsafe practices are becoming more common.

In zoos, areas are often set aside for children to pet and feed domesticated animals such as goats, sheep, and rabbits. Recently, some large public marine aquaria have introduced this practice for children so they can become familiar with sea creatures. Usually, experienced aquarium personnel remain close to the tanks to explain some of the life histories of these animals and insure that no one is injured. Though these petting tanks may provide a pleasant and educational experience, this experience could reduce or eliminate a child's innate fears of marine life while playing in the ocean, which could create risky situations.

For many years, public marine aquaria have had large sea creatures in tanks for exhibition at close range. As in the past, they continue to train marine mammals, especially porpoises and orcas (killer whales), to perform for audiences. In addition, the practice of touching, petting, feeding, and swimming with marine mammals, especially dolphins (porpoises), has been introduced. Other examples include bat ray and stingray petting pools. (The rays are reportedly debarbed.) In some aquaria, shallow small marine "touch tanks" are maintained in which sea hares, sea urchins, stinging anemones, and warty sea cucumbers can be handled. Other marine aquaria touch pools contain sharks and stingrays that can be touched, fed, and petted; some include horseshoe crabs and a variety of invertebrates. A number of aquaria will not use "touch tanks" because of the potential for inhumane treatment and possible death of the marine organisms.

Fishes

Some of the favorite marine organisms on display in aquaria are sharks and rays, usually a number of species of several families. Among bony fishes, colorful reef fishes are very popular, along with larger predatory species such as morays, snappers, groupers, and many other reef fish species. Barracudas are also attractions, partly because of their intimidating appearance. Schooling species are favorites as well, including sergeant majors, yellowtail snappers, and many species of grunts. Their well-being depends on creating an environment resembling their natural habitat, including the physical conditions in the ocean.

Marine mammals

A variety of marine mammals, including whales and dolphins, are kept in aquaria, and many are trained to perform for audiences. Others, especially dolphins *(Tursiops truncatus)* are used in therapeutic and recreational programs since they are highly intelligent. In the Florida Keys, humans can swim with dolphins in contained areas. Although some dolphins will be friendly with swimmers, a swimmer's lack of understanding of dolphin behavior could potentially lead to accidents.

In the wild, avoid close contact with dolphins since they can become unpredictable when their territory is invaded by humans. They can reach 12 feet in length and weigh up to 650 pounds, so their strike can do considerable damage and may require immediate medical attention.

Observations by scientists point out the feeding patterns used by wild dolphins to take advantage of by-products discarded at sea by fishermen. Examples include dolphins following Gulf of Mexico shrimp boats to feed on the fish and shellfish stirred up by the bottom-fishing otter trawls. Apparently the dolphins learned to distinguish between a cruising shrimp boat and one whose engines were laboring to drag the net, and they often showed up shortly after the trawling began. According to these observations, after shrimp nets are hauled aboard and unmarketable organisms thrown overboard, dolphins will follow boats, feeding on this bycatch until discarding stops. These examples of strong feeding behavior make a case against feeding wild dolphins as an attraction.

Additional Reading

Doak, W. 1989. *Human Encounters with Whales and Dolphins.* Sheridan House, Dobbs Ferry, N.Y.

Grover, W. 1989. Dolphins: One Diver's Touching Experience. *Sea Frontiers.* Internal. Oceanogr. Fndn. 35(1): 28-30.

Hillard, J. M. 1995. *Aquariums of North America: A Guidebook to Appreciating North America's Aquatic Treasures.* The Scarecrow Press, Inc. Metuchen, N.J.: 190 pp.

Livermore, B. 1991. Water Wings: Swimming with Dolphins may be the Boost Special Kids Need. *Sea Frontiers.* Internal. Oceanogr. Fndn . 37(2): 44-49, 54-55.

Perrine, D. 1989. Reef Fish Feeding: Amusement or Nuisance. *Sea Frontiers.* Internal. Oceanogr. Fndn. 35(5): 272-279.

Perrine, D. 1989. Reef Shark Attack: New Clues Raise New Questions About Why Sharks Bite People. *Sea Frontiers.* Internal. Oceanogr. Fndn. 35(1): 31-41.

Perrine, D. 1990. Jo Jo: Rogue Dolphin? *Sea Frontiers.* Internal. Oceanogr. Fndn. 36(2): 32-41.

Randall, J. E. 1968. *Caribbean Reef Fishes.* TFH Publications Neptune City, N. J.: 318 pp.

Randall, J. E. 1969. How Dangerous is the Moray Eel? *Australian Natural History.* June 1969: 177-182.

Glossary

Algae: Freshwater and marine chlorophyll-bearing plants ranging in size from a few microns to many feet in length. Single-celled, colonial, or filamentous without true leaves, roots or stems.

Amnestic shellfish poisoning (ASP): A toxin that produces memory loss and disorientation.

Arthropoda: A large group of invertebrate animals with a segmented body and jointed legs, and a hard chitinous exoskeleton; they include, among others, crustaceans, and insects.

Bacteria: Single-celled microorganisms that multiply by simple division and can be seen only by microscope. Some cause diseases in live organisms.

Bivalves: Mollusks with two shell halves or valves hinged together, such as oysters, mussels, and clams.

Branchiura: Fish lice. Taxonomic term for a crustacean class that includes crablike organisms, which are temporary ectoparasites on fishes. The genus Argulus is common on many species of fish.

Carapace: Chitinous or calcareous (bonelike) shield that covers the cephalothrax of some crustaceans. Also, the dorsal portion of a turtle shell.

Cartilage: A type of connective tissue that forms an important part of the endoskeleton of all vertebrates.

Caudal peduncle: The portion of a fish that lies between the posterior end of the anal fin and the tail base; the normally slender portion of the body that immediately precedes the tail.

Cephalothorax: In crustaceans, the body region formed by the fusion of head and thorax.

Cestode: Flat, ribbon-shaped parasitic worm.

Chitin: Horny, living substance forming the chief component of the exoskeleton of crustaceans and other invertebrates.

Chitinoclastic bacteria: Microorganisms that destroy the chitinous exoskeleton of several species of crustaceans.

Ciguatera: Nerve poisoning contracted by humans eating ciguatoxic fish. Numerous tropical fish can be affected; the poison is related to the fish's diet rather than spoilage or illness.

Coelenterata: A phylum of invertebrates that includes the jellyfish, hydroids, sea anemones, and stony and soft corals.

Columnaris disease: Disease caused by a bacterium that enters the fish through the skin and gills.

Commensalism: A form of symbiosis.

Condition Factor (Coefficient of Condition): Describes the "well being" or fatness of a fish.

Copepod: One of a subclass (Copepoda) of minute crustaceans. Some species are free-living and serve as food for many aquatic animals; other species are parasitic on the skin, scales, and gills of fish.

Cotton-wool disease: Bacterial disease of fish manifested by off-white tufts around the mouth, fins, or body.

Crustacea: A class of invertebrates belonging to the phylum Arthropoda. Crustacea are mainly aquatic and characterized by an exoskeleton of chitin divided into head, thorax, and abdomen. Examples are shrimps, lobsters, crabs, and copepods.

Decapoda: Order of crustaceans, having five pairs of legs on the thorax; includes shrimps, crabs, and lobsters.

Dermatitis: Skin inflammation.

Diatom: Microscopic unicellular or colonial algae with silica skeletons.

Digenetic trematodes: Parasitic flatworms whose life cycles usually require several hosts.

Dinoflagellates: Minute, mostly free-swimming protozoa abundant in the oceans; they are important constituents of plankton. Some species occasionally occur in large numbers, producing potent toxins that may cause "red tide," resulting in fish kills.

Dorsal: Back surface of an animal.

Dropsy: Edema; excessive fluid in cells, tissues, or body cavities of fish, caused by bacterial or viral infection.

Ecdysis: In Arthropoda, periodic shedding of the exoskeleton; molting.

Echinoids: Sea urchins and their relatives.

Ectoparasite: An organism living on the outside of another organism (the host) and dependent on the host for its metabolism, for example, leeches on the skin of fishes.

Endoparasite: An organism living inside another organism (the host) and dependent on the host for its metabolism.

Enteric redmouth: Highly infectious bacterial disease of trout and salmonids.

Epizootic: Disease attacking a large number of animals, nearly simultaneously (as an epidemic).

Erysepeloid: Refers to a human skin disease, caused when wounds become infected by bacteria from fish, and characterized by red-colored lesions.

Estuary: Bay or inlet where the ocean's tide meets the current of a freshwater river which enters the sea. (These are generally areas of high productivity.)

Euryhaline: Refers to marine organisms adaptable to a wide range of salinity.

Exotic species: An organism introduced from a different geographic region. The native range of the species is outside of the region where it has been introduced.

Exoskeleton: Exterior covering of certain animals, such as the shells of crustaceans.

Fin rot: Split, ragged fins caused by bacterial infection.

Fingerling: Young fish, larger than a fry but not an adult; usually between 0.8 and 10 inches.

Fish lice: See Branchiura

Foot: In many mollusks, a ventral structure found serving a variety of uses, including locomotion and digging.

Fry: Very young post-larval fish.

Furunculosis: Boils, skin abscesses.

Gastropods: Class of mollusks that includes whelks, slugs, and snails.

Genus: A group in the classification of organisms; subdivision of a family; taxonomic term.

Gonads: Gamete-producing reproductive organs.

Hirudinea: Leeches; parasitic or predatory annelid worms.

Host: An organism on or in which a parasite lives and from which it receives required metabolic products.

Hydrocortisone cream: Used in the treatment of inflammatory and allergic diseases.

Hydrozoa: Class of coelenterates.

Intertidal zone: Area on the foreshore between low tide and high tide.

Invertebrates: Animals without backbones.

Isopods: Small marine, freshwater, and terrestrial crustaceans, with flattened bodies and no carapace; mostly scavengers, some are parasites on fish and other crustaceans.

Larva: Immature stage of an animal that differs greatly in appearance and behavior from the adult.

Leeches: See Hirudinea.

Lesions: Sores or open wounds, may be caused by microorganisms or parasites.

Lymphocystis disease: Viral infection of fish that produces growths on fins.

Mollusks: Soft-bodied animals, mostly with calcareous shells. In some species the shell is lacking or very small.

Molt: Periodic shedding of the outer covering, such as the exoskeleton in the Arthropoda (shrimps, crabs, lobster, etc.).

Monogenetic trematodes: Ectoparasitic flatworms with hooks and suckers. Life history involves no intermediate hosts.

Mucus: Thick, slimy secretion of the mucus membranes.

Nematodes: Roundworms, which can be both free-living and parasitic.

Operculum: Gill cover; a bony covering protecting the gills of many species of fish.

Parasite: An organism that lives part or all of its life in or on another organism and is dependent on the host for its metabolism.

Pelecypod: A class of mollusks with platelike gills and compressed bodies enclosed in bivalve shells.

Pesticide: Chemical substance generally used to kill agricultural pests.

Phylum: Any of the main divisions of the animal or plant kingdom.

Plankton: Floating or drifting marine life near the ocean surface. The organisms, both plant and animal, are usually microscopic or relatively small. They float more or less passively with the currents or prevailing water movements.

Pollution: Degradation of water quality by sewage, petroleum products or other chemicals, toxic metals, pesticides, and industrial wastes which create a hazard to public health and may kill or stress aquatic organisms.

Polyp: A single individual of a colony or a solitary attached Coelenterate.

Postlarvae: Stages that resemble the juvenile but are still lacking some adult characters.

Protozoa: Single-celled animals.

Pruritic: Intense itching of the skin without eruption.

Roe: Usually refers to eggs of female fishes when still enclosed in the ovarian membrane, but in the case of sea urchins both male and female gonads are marketed and called "roe."

Salmonella: A genus of bacteria that may cause spoilage in seafood, resulting in consumer illness.

Scombroid poisoning: Caused by eating mackerels and tunas not properly refrigerated after capture. Scombrotoxin is produced by bacteria.

Secrete: To form and release a substance, such as a specified secretion from a gland.

Shellfishes: Fishery term. Aquatic invertebrates possessing a shell or exoskeleton, usually mollusks or crustaceans.

Species: A category of biological classification: a single distinct kind of animal or plant.

Sting: To prick or wound with a sharp point. Certain animals use a sharp-pointed organ to inject poison.

Suctoria: Parasitic ciliates that attack the gills of fish.

Symbiosis: Association between two species that is to the advantage of one member without seriously inconveniencing the other member. This can be in form of commensalism, mutualism, or parasitism.

Trematodes: Group of parasitic flatworms, some of which occur as parasites of aquatic animals.

Trichodina: Common ectoparasitic ciliate which may be pathogenic to aquatic organisms.

Turbidity: Cloudy condition of water, usually caused by turbulence raising sediments, including impurities such as pollutants. In the ocean, it may result from wave action stirring up bottom sediments, or from dredging operations.

Venom: Here, poison secreted by some fishes, usually introduced into the body of the victim by stinging.

Venomous: Having a poison gland or glands and able to inflict a poisonous wound by biting or stinging.

Vertebrates: Higher animals with backbones (vertebrae).

Vibrios: Here, serious bacterial pathogens of marine fishes.

Zooplankton: Usually small animals, such as crustaceans and jellyfishes, that drift with the currents. They consume other small plankton, and in turn serve as food for larger

INDEX

CP refers to the color plates in the insert.

Illustration Credits

1. *Octopus* sp. by M. Schmale

2. Stoplight Parrotfish *(Sparisoma viride)* by M. Schmale

3. Fire Worm *(Hermodice carunculata)* by S. Frink

4. Queen Conch *(Strombus gigas)* by S. Frink

5. Scrawled Cowfish *(Lactophrys quadricornis)* by S. Frink

6. Scrawled Filefish *(Aluterus scriptus)* by S. Frink

7. Spotted Morray *(Gymnothorax moringa)* by S. Frink

8. Peacock Flounder *(Bothus lunatus)* by S. Frink

9. Scorpionfish *(Scorpaena* sp.) by S. Frink

10. Yellow Goatfish *(Mullodichthys martinicus)* by S. Frink

11. High Hat *(Equetus acuminatus)* by S. Frink

12. Nassau Grouper *(Epinephelus striatus)* by S. Frink

13. Hogfish *(Lachnolaimus maximus)* by S. Frink

14. Midnight Parrotfish *(Scarus coelestinus)* by S. Frink

15. Grunts *(Haemulon* spp.) by S. Frink

16. Ocean Surgeon *(Acanthurus bahianus)* by S. Frink

17. Snook *(Centropomus undecimalis)* by S. Frink

18. Schoolmaster Snapper *(Lutjanus apodus)* by S. Frink

19. Hawksbill Turtle *(Eretmochelys imbricata)* by S. Frink

20. Great Barracuda *(Sphyraena barracuda)* by S. Frink

21. Long-spined Black Urchin *(Diadema antillarum)* by S. Frink

22. Porcupinefish *(Diodan hystrix)* by S. Frink

23. Shark *(Carcharhinus* sp.) by S. Frink

24. Blue Crab *(Callinectes sapidus)* by S. Frink

25. Fire Coral *(Millepora* sp.) by S. Frink

26. Portuguese Man-of-War *(Physalia physalis)* by S. Frink

27. American Crocodile *(Crocodylus acutus)* by S. Frink

28. King Mackerel *(Scomberomorus cavalla)* by Diane Peebles

29. Spotted Seatrout *(Cynoscion nebulosus)* by Diane Peebles

30. Striped Mullet *(Mugil cephalus)* by Diane Peebles

31. Bluefish *(Pomatomus saltatrix)* by Diane Peebles

32. Crevalle Jack *(Caranx hippos)* by Diane Peebles

33. Gafftopsail Catfish *(Bagre marinus)* by Diane Peebles

34. Southern Stingray *(Dasyatis americana)* by Diane Peebles

Here are some other books from Pineapple Press on related topics. For a complete catalog, write to Pineapple Press, P.O. Box 3889, Sarasota, Florida 34230-3889, or call (800) 746-3275. Or visit our website at www.pineapplepress.com.

Common Coastal Birds of Florida and the Caribbean by David W. Nellis. This comprehensive guide reveals 72 of the most common birds found along the coasts of Florida and the islands to the south. Includes abundant information on each bird's nesting, feeding, mating, and migrating habits, as well as more than 250 color photos that show many features of these birds never before so fully illustrated. (hb & pb)

Florida Magnificent Wilderness by James Valentine and D. Bruce Means. A visual journey through some of the most precious wild areas in the state, presenting the breathtaking beauty preserved in state lands, parks, and natural areas. Valentine has used his camera to record environmental art images of the state's remote wilderness places. Dr. D. Bruce Means has written the detailed captions and main text, "Florida's Rich Biodiversity." Each section of the book has an introduction written by a highly respected Florida writer and conservationist. (hb)

Florida's Birds, 2nd Edition: A Field Guide and Reference by David S. Maehr and Herbert W. Kale II. Illustrated by Karl Karalus. Now with color throughout, this new edition includes 30 new species accounts. Each bird is illustrated 3 times—with the species account, in the index listing, and on a plate with similar species to aid in identification. Sections on bird study, feeding, and habitats; threatened and endangered species; exotic species; and bird conservation. (pb)

Poisonous Plants and Animals of Florida and the Caribbean by David W. Nellis. An illustrated guide to the characteristics, symptoms, and treatments for more than 300 species of poisonous plants and toxic animals. (hb)

Priceless Florida by Ellie Whitney, Bruce Means, and Anne Rudloe. An extensive guide (432 pages, 800 color photos) to the incomparable ecological riches of this unique region, presented in a way that will appeal to young and old, layperson and scientists. Complete with maps, charts, species lists. (hb & pb)

Seashore Plants of South Florida and the Caribbean by David W. Nellis. A color guide to the flora of nearshore environments, including complete charac istics of each plant as well as ornamental, medicinal, ecological, and o aspects. Suitable for both backyard gardeners and serious naturalists. (pb)